Nurse! Nurse!

A Student Nurse's Story

Jimmy Frazier

Constable · London

Constable & Robinson Ltd
3 The Lanchesters
162 Fulham Palace Road
London W6 9ER
www.constablerobinson.com

First published in the UK by Constable,
an imprint of Constable & Robinson Ltd, 2011

A copy of the British Library Cataloguing in
Publication data is available from the British Library

ISBN: 978-1-84529-395-6

Printed and bound in the EU

1 3 5 7 9 10 8 6 4 2

ACKNOWLEDGEMENTS

Thank you to all my nursing colleagues – fellow students, mentors, teachers – and to my many patients. I salute you all, even Mr Temple. Vicks, Catherine, SP, Laura – I couldn't have made it without you.

On the writing front, Andreas, Barbara, Sylvia and Matt have all been stars. Thanks, too, to Maria, my inspiring muse.

My book is not academic at all, but I would like to thank the following authors for their hard-won research and insights: Neel Burton, Sebastian Faulks, Oliver James, Oliver Sacks and Irvin Yalom.

I am, as always, humbled and grateful for the continual support of my family and friends – you know who you are! – and, above all, to Poppin, my faraway angel.

With love
to my sisters, Elizabeth and Frances

NOTE ON THE TEXT

So, is this account true? Well, yes, in that much of what happened in these pages is based on my student nursing experiences. And no, in that all the characters are composites and have had their names and identities completely changed to protect confidentiality. Jimmy Frazier is also a pseudonym.

Chapter 1

STARTING OVER

First up was the interview – or in NHS speak: 'Suitability Test'.

I put on a dark suit, a pair of polished black Doc Martens and pinned a Remembrance Day poppy to my lapel. It was the smartest I'd looked in years.

At the hospital reception I was asked: 'Whose father are you?'

'Nobody's!' I harrumphed, and explained I was one of the nursing candidates.

'Oh, sorry, sir,' said the blond supervisor, peering at me through trendy, blue-rimmed glasses. 'We don't get many applicants looking like you.'

'George Clooney types?' I suggested, though Wayne Rooney was probably more accurate.

'You wish, sir! I mean middle-aged men wearing a suit and tie.'

In the 'Selection Day' room there were fourteen other candidates. It was a large, light room, midway up a tower block. The only feature, other than desks and chairs, was a shelf of blood pressure machines that resembled an army of midget aliens.

The other candidates were all young women between the ages of eighteen and twenty-five. I was the only man and the eldest by comfortably a decade, although at times that morning it felt more like several geological eras. Many of the girls wore tracksuits or denim. Four or five were zombied out, listening to iPods. The only sounds were the *slop, slop* of chewed gum and some distant church bells.

I was sitting next to a teenager who, unlike most of the others, was immaculately dressed in a blue top decorated with seahorses. Her pretty, freckled face was pale as a candle and pinched with nerves.

'Don't worry,' I said, trying to relax her. 'It's only a basic Maths and English test.'

'God, I'm so nervous,' she replied, biting her lip. 'All I ever wanted is to be a children's nurse. Ever since I was little.'

Elsa told me about her volunteer work in hospitals over the school holidays, looking after her ailing grandfather and gaining a First Aid certificate. She'd also written a project on Edith Cavell, the heroic wartime nurse shot by the Nazis after helping allied soldiers escape from Belgium.

I felt like a fraud by comparison. All I'd done in preparation was watch the boxed set of *Grey's Anatomy*, perhaps the least authentic hospital show ever aired on television. *'Nurse! Nurse! It's Dr Implausible here, we've got a dozen earthquake victims, a wounded deer and a woman who thinks she's Abraham Lincoln. Oh, and I'll see you in the locker room after you're done, you saucy minx.'*

My own experience had been far from medical. I'd spent years odd-jobbing: working on farms, in bars and restaurants, teaching English to the Chinese. I didn't have one member of my immediate family – past or present – who had worked in medicine and I'd never even seen a dead body – except on *Grey's Anatomy*. 'What the hell am I doing here?' I thought to myself, not for the first time that morning.

'God, I'm just so nervous,' Elsa repeated. She was becoming increasingly uptight, tapping her foot against her desk.

'Don't panic,' I said. 'You'll be fine.'

A side door swung open and in shot a small, bearded man

with a rucksack the size of a straw bale. He strutted to the front of the class and cavalierly discarded his load.

'Good morning,' he said, scanning us all. 'My name is Mr Temple.' He smiled menacingly. 'I'm here to tell you that you are mine for the next three years. All mine!' Elsa nodded enthusiastically. 'Turn off those iPods!'

A couple of the girls begrudgingly ripped out their earplugs.

'Now listen carefully,' Mr Temple continued, while prowling between desks. 'You might have friends who are studying something nice and soft. Something like history, or art, or media. Pah! They get most of the summer off and a long break at Easter and Christmas.' At this point he raised his voice. 'But *you*, you won't. You get about five weeks. The rest of the time you are in the wards or studying. In other words – you are mine! All mine! Am I clear?'

Elsa nodded even more enthusiastically. I prayed she never got kidnapped by a cult as she would be brainwashed in no time.

'Maybe you like playing sport at weekends,' added Mr Temple, 'perhaps singing in a choir, salsa dancing or, God help us, shopping. Well, that's fine. But nursing will come first. OK? If it doesn't, then feel free to leave now. The door is there.' He stabbed a finger in its direction. 'So go now. *Go!*' Elsa looked miserably at the door, her eyes wide as saucers. I was making a Herculean effort not to laugh. If Mr Temple said, 'You are mine. All mine!' one more time, I felt sure I would.

'Did you know the NHS is the largest employer in Europe?' barked Mr Temple. 'And the third largest employer in the world. Did you know? Did *you?*' Elsa shook her head. I joined her this time. I decided I probably shouldn't get kidnapped by a cult either. 'You are in a privileged position, every one of you. It costs over £11,000 a year to train a nurse, so don't come expecting an easy ride. Every year there are high dropout rates.'

Mr Temple banged his fist on a desk. Elsa flinched. 'Nursing is not all about helping nice little children. Oh, no! It's a hard

3

job – you will have to deal with blood, tears, abuse, horrible parents, fear and death. So if it's not for you, get out now. Right now. Go on, *out!*' The man really was a charmer. I sensed Elsa was about to pass out – she'd been expecting a Maths test, for heaven's sake.

'But, trust me, all of you,' Mr Temple softened his voice. 'If you make it, you will have one of the most rewarding jobs in the world. I really mean that.' He smiled, a genuinely warm smile this time. 'And I hope you will all make it.'

Blimey, he had turned into the Nurse Whisperer. Elsa was now beaming with a wattage that verged on celestial.

'Right! First the English test, then Maths,' snapped Mr Temple, ruining the moment. I'd have to get used to this Good Nurse, Bad Nurse routine.

The English test was fine but, having not even looked at an equation for twenty years, I struggled with the Maths. Elsa had clearly breezed through both, and seemed relaxed for the first time that morning.

'Right, next we're going to have a debate,' said Mr Temple, pulling out a handful of cardboard signs from his rucksack. He explained that on each of the signs was a question. For example: Are celebrities bad for our health? Are nurses too posh to wash?

Mr Temple told us to pull our chairs into a circle facing each other. We were then each handed a cardboard sign. Mine read: Should alcohol be banned? And Elsa's: Is the media too powerful? Elsa looked nervous again.

The idea was that each of us should speak for five minutes on our subject, but that others could join in, too. First up was a very assured West Indian girl talking about celebrities. All was going fine until near the end when she started talking about George Best.

'So, tell me,' interrupted Mr Temple abruptly, 'should George Best have been allowed another liver?'

'No,' I said. This was something I felt strongly about. 'He was given one liver, then carried on boozing. Why should he have another?'

'Because he was a football legend,' argued a brunette with a hint of an Irish accent. 'And what are you going to do, just let him die?'

'He was a washed-out playboy,' I said. 'So many people deserved a liver more than he did. Sure, he was a genius once, but he'd had his chance.'

'You're supposed to be a nurse, supposed to care,' fumed the brunette, not unreasonably. 'There were personal reasons for his drinking.'

'I didn't want him to die, I liked him,' I stressed. 'But there aren't many livers available. I think someone else should have had it, that's all.'

Oh no, this wasn't going well at all. I'd wanted to passionately express my views, but had come across like a tabloid pundit.

The rest of the talks went smoothly enough. I interjected here and there, trying to sound a bit more touchy-feely, and a bit less like George Best's assassin. During my talk: Should alcohol be banned? I stressed that it shouldn't – partly because prohibition had been a disaster in 1920s America and partly because it was a denial of our human rights, but mostly because I liked a pint now and then. I was challenged by a feisty, bespectacled girl who raged about alcohol being the 'devil's juice'. This made me feel a bit less hard line.

But I was worried about Elsa. She hadn't said a word. Her topic hadn't come up yet. When it did, she looked close to tears. She read out in a quavering voice: 'Is the media too powerful?' then dried up completely. Several of us tried to help her out, but she was stiff with nerves, utterly mute. Her head slumped down and her eyes welled up. She didn't say another word and before long the final talk had been presented and we were free to go.

I accompanied Elsa to the bus stop. She burst into tears as soon as we left the building.

'I didn't say anything,' she said, her breath smoky in the cold air. 'They'll never select me. I've failed. I'll never be a nurse.'

'Don't worry,' I tried to reassure her. 'It probably doesn't matter. Some of us said far too much. You did well in the written tests. You'll be fine.'

'No, I'm out,' said Elsa, rummaging in her handbag for a tissue. 'I'm sure of it.'

Sadly, she was probably right. And yet, out of all of us, I sensed she was the most naturally caring, and certainly wasn't too posh to wash. It seemed so unfair that a nineteen-year-old's ability to nurse was being judged on whether she could tell us: Is the media too powerful? Something even Jeremy Paxman might struggle with.

But maybe Elsa was just too nice. I had read about nurses having to endure 'the tyranny of niceness'. About how they are supposed to be constantly full of smiles and good will towards everyone at all times. Elsa had this ability in abundance. And yet, early in my course I realised nurses also had to be resilient. They had to stand up for themselves, whether in front of patients and their families, or fellow health professionals. At times they would witness tragic incidents, verbal abuse, and long hours. They needed to be strong. Yet wasn't there room for gentle nurses such as Elsa, and tougher ones such as Mr Temple?

For all Mr Temple's belligerence, I soon realised it had been for a reason. He was right to tell us it was going to be hard, and that we wouldn't have much time for other things. He was even right to stress: 'You are mine. All mine.' And he was right to tell us it could be the most rewarding job in the world, too.

'I'll see you at the hospital,' I told Elsa, who had now dried her tears. She smiled, a fragile but dignified smile, and walked on to her bus. I never saw her or any of the others again. Oh, except Mr Temple, of course.

To celebrate being accepted as a trainee nurse I joined Jake and Bill, two of my oldest friends, at our local, The Rising Sun. Jake, a teacher of English as a foreign language, was dressed in a blue poncho.

'What's this, Jakey-Boy?' said Bill, shaking dry his umbrella. 'Casual Friday?'

'You know every day's casual with me, Bill,' replied Jake. 'But I've got a Mexican in my class this week, so I'm making him feel at home.'

'Feel at home!' said Bill. 'You look like Clint Eastwood in drag.'

In contrast to Jake's outré dress sense, Bill was wearing a beige suit, the sort of garment diplomats wear in films. He worked all hours in the human resources department of a construction company to support his ever-expanding family.

'Take a look at this, Jimmy,' said Bill, slapping down a newspaper. MRSA – SHOULD WE BLAME NURSES? blazed the headline.

'I'd be worried if you were my nurse, Jimmy,' said Jake. 'Your personal hygiene was never very good when we shared a house together.'

'That was then, this is now, Jake. I even floss my teeth sometimes these days.'

Bill pointed triumphantly at another article further into the paper. VIOLENT ATTACKS ON NURSING SOARING.

'Are you really sure you want to do this, amigo?' said Jake, slapping me on the back. 'Let's face it, you're hardly Mother Teresa are you? All this sudden worthiness sounds like a midlife crisis to me.'

'Don't worry,' I said. 'I'm ready. I've read the articles, too.' And I had, every one of them: NO JOBS FOR NEW NURSES; NURSING IN THE UK – NO THANKS; and NURSES ANGRY WITH THE GOVERNMENT. The list was endless.

'I just don't get it,' said Jake. 'All those negative headlines but didn't Tony Blair just boast it's the best year ever for the NHS?'

'What bollocks!' said Bill, crunching on a pork scratching. In his other hand he cradled a pint of Guinness. Without the recent smoking ban, he'd have had a Marlboro in his mouth, too.

'It's not all bad,' I said. 'Nurses' starting salaries have almost doubled over the last decade.'

'Nurses should get paid well,' said Bill. 'I read that the NHS now costs us almost 100 billion pounds a year. One hundred billion pounds!' Bill slapped his paunch in protest. 'That's a sum so bloody huge even Cristiano Ronaldo wouldn't turn up his nose at it.'

I stressed that the NHS statistics weren't all rotten. Patient deaths from cancer and heart disease were both down, and the average life expectancy in the UK was now nearly a whopping eighty years old.

'Oh, great,' said Jake. 'So the fact Bruce Forsyth is still dancing and David Attenborough still hugging gorillas is all down to the NHS.'

'Don't be so cynical,' I said. 'The NHS has its faults, sure. But it gives free health care to the country. We should be grateful. It's a national treasure!'

'Was a national treasure,' said Jake, with as much gravitas as a man in a blue poncho could muster. 'It now spends all its billions on managers.'

'But it needs managers,' said Bill. 'Just not as many. And only medically savvy ones who don't charge through the nose.'

'Like you do, Bill,' I said. 'And if you keep troughing pork fat like that you'll need the NHS before you hit forty.'

'Ooooh, matron, give me a break.' Bill winked at me. 'I make no excuses. I'm a fat businessman – get over it.'

'Florence, here,' Jake said, pointing at me, 'is right, Bill. You need to take more care of yourself. You're plump as a goose.' Being a stick-thin, rock-climbing, tofu muncher, Jake had every right to criticise Bill – but he could sound horribly smug.

'I know I'm a nurse in waiting,' I stressed. 'But could we cut down on the "oooh matron" and Florence jibes.'

So far people had reacted very differently towards my decision to be a nurse. My family and female friends – with the exception of Jess, my girlfriend – tended to bathe me in angelic glory and proudly announce: 'Jimmy's training to be a nurse you know, isn't that *lovely/noble/scary as hell.*' (The last comment was from Jess.) Many of my male friends, however, teased me relentlessly. They jested about bedpans, sensible shoes and Ann Summers suspenders. Their image of nurses seemed to veer wildly from saintly Florence Nightingale types to pouty temptresses such as Abby in *ER*.

To be fair, by starting my nurse training in my thirties, I was smashing the three golden rules of hospital soaps – namely that nurses should be one: female; two: young; and three: gorgeous. Yet one in ten nurses is now male, compared to only a handful during the birth of the NHS more than sixty years ago. In fact, there are now more male nurses than ever before with numbers steadily on the up.

Sadly, this encouraging statistic failed to stop the likes of Jake and Bill milking all the stereotypes. And by last orders that evening they were at it again.

'Hey, Bill, listen up!' Jake cupped his hand to his ear. 'It's Jimmy's song on the duke box.' In the background I could hear Robbie Williams breaking into the opening lines of 'Angels'. At the chorus they both serenaded me with a horribly off-key duet.

'And through it all, *he* offers me protection, a lot of love and affection, whether I'm right or wrong . . . '

'Please, guys, we're going to get kicked out,' I pleaded. 'You sound like Keith Richards drowning . . . '

'DuhDuhDuhDuhDuuuu . . . DuhDuhDuhDuhDuhnaaa-naaaaaaah . . . '

'Enough, you plonkers!'

'Lighten up, Jimmy,' said Jake, as he drained his pint. 'Worse things happen at sea. At least we didn't sing "Sisters Are Doing It For Themselves".'

On the first day of nursing school I arrived in good time at the assembly hall. Watching my fellow students, many of them shouldering backpacks – their faces part anxiety, part hope – I was reminded of refugees arriving in a new land.

Our group – about 150 in all – was a complex cultural stew. Voices from Africa, the West Indies, Canada, France, Eastern Europe and South America, not to mention Hackney and Huddersfield, swirled around, creating a babel that sounded as strange and rich as a flock of tropical birds.

We varied greatly in age, too. It was safe to say a few students had just left school – one girl even wore pigtails with red bows as if she'd just skipped out of *Grange Hill* – while at the other end of the scale were a few silver surfers, well into their forties and even fifties.

We really were the most incredible jumble. To my right sat Tola, a chatty Jamaican mother of three, with a Walnut Whip hairdo held in place by a lacquer so strong not even a tornado would ruffle it. And to my left was a sturdy, middle-aged man called Kiko, bald as a billiard ball, who had spent time in the Senegalese army. In front of us sat an elegant Muslim girl in a black headdress next to an exuberant Scot called Laura, a former aerobics teacher with a nose stud. Nursing clearly acted as a crucible to all ages, races, faiths – and hairdos.

Tola and Laura were both studying to be adult nurses. Adult nurses made up the lion's share of the assembly, and were mostly young women in their twenties. Kiko, however, was studying mental health – a branch of nursing that radically boosted the number of men and older students in the profession. It seemed children's nurses were the smallest group; in fact I had yet to meet one.

The assembly hall was huge, cold and dusty. There were no desks to write on, so we poised our notebooks on our laps, like journalists at a press conference.

Before the class started, a pigeon that had been roosting on the hall's roof beams began flapping around above us. A man in blue overalls appeared with a window pole. He tried chivvying the startled creature, but it only flew to a fresh perch, causing lots of cheering and whooping from the class.

'Quiet!' snapped a familiar voice.

And then, with the authority of Moses parting the Red Sea, Mr Temple walked in. The hall immediately hushed. Even the pigeon stopped cooing. What was it about this man, other than that he looked a bit like a Bond villain (the one with the white cat, I think, rather than the one with three nipples or the killer top hat)? Accompanying Mr Temple was a splendidly upright lady with a neat, black bob and the warmest of smiles. Tola told me she recognised her. She was known as Super Nurse, writer of many text books on nursing and something of a legend.

'Good morning, everyone,' said Super Nurse, beaming. 'Welcome to the Grand Hall.'

'Otherwise known as the Not So Grand Hall,' mumbled Mr Temple.

'It's a joy to see so many of you keen to become nurses,' said Super Nurse. 'The best profession there is.' Mr Temple rolled his eyes at this point. It was clear these two were going to be a great double act. Super Nurse as Tigger, Mr Temple as a much angrier version of Eeyore.

Super Nurse then proceeded to give us a half-hour barn-stormer of a speech. If this had been a party political conference, she would have won several standing ovations. Like Mr Temple, she did not shy from the profession's tougher aspects. She even confessed that she had very nearly given up in her final year of nurse training, tired and disillusioned after too many night shifts and battling with her overdraft.

Heavens above, I thought, if this human dynamo nearly threw in the towel, what hope have the rest of us? But Super Nurse dwelt on the positive, too — the soul-charging satisfaction of doing a job that improved people's lives every day.

'Whenever times are tough,' advised Super Nurse, with evangelical zeal, 'think of the good you are doing. Unlike some jobs, nursing is never trivial. You are helping the sick, the vulnerable. Is there a more rewarding job than this? I don't think so. Thank you and good luck.'

Super Nurse received a huge cheer and left us all on a high, basking in her positive aura. Mr Temple then took to the stage. Here we go, I thought, from the sublime to the sanctimonious. But, this time there wasn't to be a single 'You are mine!' It was all low-key practical stuff, with Mr Temple explaining the events of the day such as picking up uniforms and distributing timetables. Then, just as we were about to leave, he couldn't resist one final pep talk.

'You are the standard bearers of the new generation!' shouted Mr Temple. 'So don't let yourselves down. But more importantly – don't let me down!' He softened his tone. 'Many of you here will not make it through the next three years. You will fall by the wayside. You simply will not survive.' Good God, what was this? The eve of Agincourt?

'But remember, if you're struggling,' Mr Temple gestured to us all, 'and, trust me, you will struggle, remember we are here to support you. Every! Single! Step! Of! The! Way!' Another cheer erupted, almost as good as the one for Super Nurse.

'Now shut up and collect your uniforms,' snapped Mr Temple. 'And someone get that bloody pigeon out of here.'

Later, I met some of my fellow children's nurses. According to a list given to us by Mr Temple there were a dozen of us, all women except for me and a man called Chips, an Irish photographer.

Chips was the first of the group I came across. I bumped into him at the uniform fitting as I tried on my blue trousers and white tunic. I also had a badge that proudly proclaimed: JIMMY FRAZIER – STUDENT NURSE.

'Hey, it's Gordon Ramsay's little brother,' said Chips, pointing at me. To be fair the male nurse's uniform – especially the white-buttoned tunic – did make me look a bit like a chef.

Chips sported a pork-pie hat and heavy, black-framed glasses. He was about my age, perhaps a bit older. He told me that his photography work – everything from weddings to war zones – was drying up and he wanted something more stable. One of his nieces had needed heart surgery recently and the high standard of care she had received at an NHS hospital had inspired him to become a children's nurse.

During lunch break, Chips and I perused the text books at the college shop. Here we met two more of our group – Jana, a bright, rangy-limbed Bermudan girl who used to work in IT and Vicky, a boisterous Essex teenager, fresh out of school. Jana was elegantly dressed in black with a spangly, Boho necklace while Vicky sported crucifix earrings, ripped jeans and a face full of mischief. They were both ranting about the cost of books.

'How am I supposed to buy paperbacks worth twenty quid?' Vicky said, running her finger along the book spines. 'I can barely afford to pay my rent.'

'Same here,' agreed Jana. 'Even my room in the nursing hall is over sixty quid a week.'

I realised how lucky I was to be living in my own flat and without an overdraft. Chips was in a similar position to me, but for many students – especially the younger ones – money was a huge concern. Their annual bursary – around £7,000 – was their lifeline.

But Vicky and Jana had the edge on us oldies when it came to technology. Chips and I wouldn't have known a Power Point presentation if it hit us full-beam in the face. And neither of us had studied subjects such as biology, maths and essay writing since our teens. For this reason I badly needed a basic biology book and was eyeing up one called *The Body – A Duffer's Guide*.

'All I remember about biology from school days,' I said, pulling out the book, 'is that a man's body is 90 per cent water.'

'A man's body is only about 60 per cent water, actually,' Jana corrected me. 'And a woman's body 5 per cent less. Women have more body fat than men, though.'

'Where do men store their extra water, then?' asked Vicky.

'Probably their brains,' said Jana.

Apart from a basic biology primer, I also wanted a more personal book on nursing. Not a text book, but a blow-by-blow account of what it is like to be a nurse today, of life on the wards. Incredibly, there didn't seem to be one. There were stretcherloads of books by other health professionals – surgeons, doctors, paramedics – and several couchloads by therapists, with titles such as *Oedipus Revisited* and *How to Make Somebody Fall in Love with You in 10 Minutes: or Less*! – but not one contemporary nursing book.

Considering there are more nurses than any other health professionals in the NHS, and the NHS employs over a million staff, this was an arresting fact. The only nursing memoirs on show were Florence Nightingale's dispatches from the Crimea. Groundbreaking, sure – but over 150 years old.

'Of course there are no nursing memoirs,' Vicky told me, decisively. 'Nurses are far too busy to ponce about writing books.'

She had a point. The nurses I met always seemed active, practical people. They wanted to crack on and care for the sick, frail, mentally ill, and when not dashing about doing this they liked to gossip and eat biscuits. Finding their inner muse was understandably low on their priority list.

Eventually, I bought a basic biology book and a discounted copy of *The Motorcycle Diaries* by Che Guevara, which I found in the history section – Mr Temple would not have approved. I told Chips that as Che Guevara had trained to be a doctor in his early life, this was my excuse for buying his diary.

'Rubbish,' said Jana, reading the front cover, which showed Che on his Norton 500. 'You bought it so that if the nursing doesn't work out, you can become a revolutionary.'

'Well, the hours are probably better,' mused Vicky. 'Wages, too. And you get to grow the coolest beard in history.'

In sharp contrast to Che Guevara's beard, that afternoon we confronted the two least cool beards in history. These belonged to a pair of St John Ambulance workers – Rob and Robbie – our manual handling teachers.

It was hard to tell Rob and Robbie apart. Both had equal amounts of jungly, grey-flecked facial hair and matching blue jumpers with elbow patches. They resembled Arctic explorers who'd just returned from the Pole, although judging by the size of their paunches they had tucked into too many walrus suppers en route. In fact, Rob and Robbie were so hard to tell apart that Vicky decided we should simply call them The Beards.

The Beards' class was the first to bring our group together.

Other than Chips, Jana, Vicky and myself there were two very polite, slightly anxious Muslim girls enshrouded in black (Hadia and Shima); a Zimbabwean mother of four with a booming laugh (Sheena); a serene Ghanaian woman, who had a degree in marketing (Coco); a Somali girl with an equatorial girth disguised by beautiful, swirling robes (Ola), and a tiny, smiley girl from Cameroon who was reading a Mills and Boon romance (Mayla).

The Beards were veteran teachers blessed with a confident, easy banter. They had their 'How to Lift' lesson down to a tee.

Robbie (or maybe Rob) was first up. We have 206 bones in our body, he told us while primping his side-burns, and of these, our spinal vertebrae are the most crucial for lifting.

'And did you know,' said Rob (or Robbie), 'nursing is perhaps the most dangerous profession of all for knackering your back?'

Vicky quickly raised her hand: 'What about weightlifters?'

'Or sheep shearers?' I said.

'Or builders?' suggested Sheena.

Rob looked at us, unfazed, and said that nurses historically had more back injuries than builders. He said he'd never tried sheep shearing or weightlifting himself – 'I leave all the heavy lifting to the missus' – but he imagined both professions required strong backs to start with. He stressed that nurses had to lift patients of all shapes and sizes – even children's nurses, such as us, would have to deal with some hefty teenagers.

Nowadays though, Robbie assured us, nurses didn't really need to lift at all – thanks to hoists, which we would be taught how to use later.

'In fact,' Robbie said, 'the only movement you need on the wards now is this . . . ' He slightly bent his knees, parted his legs and gently rocked back and forth. 'And that's it,' he said. 'No need to tense muscles, no need to twist your back. Just like a reed in the breeze.'

At this stage all hell broke loose. Some of the students had recently worked on wards as volunteers or health care assistants and insisted they had done lots of manual hefting.

'Listen up!' said Rob, raising his hands. 'If any of you are asked to lift a patient manually you needn't do it. Simple as that. Just call me and I'll speak to the ward manager. I'll write my number on the board.'

I was impressed by this gesture and could see it was genuine but I also knew there was a huge difference between what Rob was teaching in the class, and the reality of the wards.

Clearly if a patient fell to the floor in a hospital and no hoist was available we couldn't simply leave them. If we refused to help – 'Sorry, Matron, there's no way I'm lifting *anyone*, Rob said so, OK!' – surely we would be laughed out of town. It would be like an army cadet refusing to do an assault course. 'Sorry, Sarge, in school we were told not to climb ropes unless we really had to. I'm texting my health and safety adviser.'

But Rob did have a very good point. 'You only get one spine so be careful,' he said, a biscuit vanishing into the wilderness of his beard. 'Damage it and your career is over.'

As we finished the lesson early Robbie asked us all to briefly give our reasons for wanting to become a nurse. Chips mentioned his visits to see his niece in hospital while Jana had been inspired by her doctor father. Others had helped care for family members – a parent with dementia, a sister with autism – and some had been won over by volunteer work. Hadia, with winning clarity, simply told us: 'I was born to nurse.'

Fortunately, the class finished before it was my turn. I knew I would have trouble explaining my reasons for nursing as eloquently as my colleagues. In truth, I was still working them out.

Chapter 2

GROWING PAINS

My first taste of working in a hospital was as a schoolboy. At the time this sparked in me an overwhelming urge – never, ever, to become a nurse.

One summer holiday I had volunteered to help out at a hospital near to my sister's flat in south London. This all sounds very noble. It wasn't. During term time I'd been caught drinking a flagon of snakebite with some mates on the school playing fields. The volunteer work was simply punishment for my indiscreet boozing.

I approached the hospital with the idea of doing some gardening or other such physical labour. As a boy in my mid-teens, with no interest in medicine, I didn't want to go anywhere near a patient. And so, sod's law, I was immediately posted to what was called in those politically incorrect days a geriatric ward.

I still remember it now. The complicated smells of bleach, cabbage, floor polish and old people. I remember the patients lining the ward walls, facing each other, many of them hunched in wheelchairs. I remember their pale, weary faces, almost translucent in the morning sun. I remember groans of pain, and occasional bursts of laughter; pop music forever playing softly in the background. And I remember the nurses. They whirled around the ward dressing wounds, dishing out pills, washing limbs, changing sheets, smiling, dancing. A posse of fairy-tale dervishes in blue.

At first I struggled badly. Of course I'd been to hospitals before – a fractured tibia, a smashed collar bone, the usual youthful prangs – but only ever to A & E. Never somewhere like this. A place where people needed help with absolutely everything. Everything! Waking, washing, feeding, moving, even breathing.

My own grandparents – barring a grandfather who had died when I was tiny – were all hale and hearty back then. But here, among these exhausted souls, I felt as if I'd landed on another planet. I hated it. All around was the whiff of decay, the shadow of death.

The nurses broke me in gently. On the first day I took several patients out for walks in the garden. It was a quadrangle of green, studded with statues and fountains. Doves cooed in the yew trees. I talked to the patients as I steered them around, but only a few answered.

On one such walk, an ancient fellow, frail as something newly hatched, began wailing – 'Ayyyahhh'. I ushered him back to the ward in terror.

The nurses just laughed. 'Mr Jenkins always makes a bit of noise,' they said. 'Don't worry, he's fine. Keep him moving.'

At lunchtime I helped feed the patients. I would spoon mouthfuls of mush into wrinkled, quivering mouths and wipe any drool from cheeks and chins. Some of the diners would smile and thank me, some would remain quiet, and others would fall fast asleep. The nurses chattered away, ever jovial, telling patients about their day or what they'd seen on telly. I found their animation impressive but rather pointless; surely not even a starburst of fireworks would lighten up that sorry place.

On my first afternoon I helped dress the leg ulcer of a patient named Mr Riley – most patients were called by their surname then. Mr Riley was suffering from advanced Parkinson's disease.

His limbs shook and flinched and his head nodded all over the place. Mrs Riley was also in the room; a stout, benign-faced woman, hovering over her husband.

All I had to do was help keep Mr Riley still while the nurse, a sunny, fiftyish African woman named Shula, swabbed the ulcer. I still remember the moment Shula pulled off Mr Riley's bandage. The wound yawned up at us, pale and damp, with a crust of blackened blood. The bandage was hard to pull off, as if feeding on his skin. The stench was excruciating, and I struggled not to retch.

Shula dabbed away, singing softly to Mr Riley, as he moaned. I kept hold of his legs and watched as Shula applied a sheaf of gauze with graceful, well-practised moves. When she was done, Shula dropped the soiled swabs on to a tray, and ripped off her surgical gloves. She asked me to stay and keep Mr Riley company, as his wife was about to leave.

I sat by Mr Riley's bed. He soon fell asleep. After a while the old man's breathing stopped for so long I feared him dead, but then he gasped wildly, as if he'd had a sudden epiphany. His rheumy eyes focused on me, full of wonder and panic.

'Mary?' he asked, his grip tightening on my hand. 'I want Mary.' I assured Mr Riley his wife would be in tomorrow. I'd been told she visited daily. 'But you're not my wife. I want Mary. Mary! MARY!'

Mr Riley lunged towards me, half slipping off the bed on to his bad leg. He was wired to a drip and I was worried his tubes might rip out. I supported him as best I could. The pain from his ulcer must have been appalling but he seemed oblivious. 'MARY! MARY!' By this stage I was holding on to Mr Riley's wrists. They felt tight as hawsers. As he struggled he began to weep.

'It's OK, Mr Riley,' I pleaded, utterly out of my depth. 'Please, Mr Riley, it's really OK, please don't cry. Your wife will visit soon.' Nothing would placate him. I shouted for Shula.

Within seconds Shula ripped back the cubicle curtain, and helped me prop Mr Riley back on the bed. He was moaning his wife's name repeatedly like a desperate mantra. The noise was awful: something not of this world. Shula stood over him, relaxed as ever, and stroked his forehead, whispering to Mr Riley as if he were a child. She upped his morphine and soon he was quiet and, before long, asleep.

'Poor man,' I said, washing my hands in a basin by the bed. 'He really misses his wife.'

'Oh, he's one of the lucky ones,' whispered Shula, watching Mr Riley's uneven breathing. 'At least he has a wife to visit him. That lady there,' she gestured to a powdery old woman in the next bed, 'her son lives just down the road but he can't face seeing her. Wants to remember her before she was all weak and muddled up.' Shula shook her head. 'Others have no one at all to visit. Lonely as wolves they are. You'll see things here, darling, that will break your heart.'

I asked Shula how she could do this every day. She laughed and playfully punched my arm. 'Oh, Jimmy,' she said. 'How much you have to learn. Your problem is how you are looking at them.' She made a gesture towards Mr Riley. 'You ain't seeing the human being, just the body. Some of these old folks here had lives you wouldn't believe.' She pointed to the opposite side of the ward. 'Now, Gillian, over there, she's swum the English Channel. Check out the photo by her bed sometime. She's a treasure.'

She went on to tell me about Mr Grantham, who wore a head bandage and had fought in the Great War and Mr Simms who once played the violin in some big-time orchestra but was now addled with dementia. Then there was snow-haired, silent Miss Parsons, an ex-missionary, who had a scrapbook of photos of herself as a carefree adventuress in the jungles of Indonesia.

Shula moved towards me, lowering her voice even more. 'And don't forget Mr Riley here, he's a dark horse, you know.

21

Mrs Riley is his fourth wife.' She nudged my arm and shrieked with laughter. 'Bet you wouldn't have guessed that, hey, Jimmy!'

In those early days, as a schoolboy on the wards, I just couldn't hack it, seeing so many patients so utterly alone. Of course, there were those with doting families, who visited regularly and left sweets and flowers and photos of grandchildren. But other patients never had so much as a Get Well card grace their bedside, let alone a bunch of grapes.

I was from a huge, chaotic family, full of the usual feuds, comedy and love. There were loads of us – we bred like kangaroos – and that somehow made me feel safe. Yet there, in that fit-to-burst ward, were dozens of aged souls, bedbound and scared, left with nobody. Through my teenage eyes, yet to confront loneliness, let alone death, it seemed the worst thing in the world.

'Hardly anyone writes to old people,' Shula told me one morning. 'Let alone crazy, old people.' And she was right.

It was the nurses who kept me going. They were a tight, intimate and upbeat bunch. They gave each other raucous nicknames – Charlotte the Harlot, Juicy Lucy, Betty Boo – and, over lunch, would gossip away with cheerful indiscretion: 'My hubby couldn't get it up last night, needs to eat more bananas,' or 'I was at it all weekend, now I'm walking round like a bloody cowboy.' They could be bitchy and cruel, but when one of them was in trouble everyone would rally. While I was there, one of the sisters, a quiet, no-nonsense woman called Beverly, lost her husband to cancer. Almost all the nurses attended the funeral and wrote the most sensitive messages on her card. It was as if their nursing – so hard to explain to others – gave them membership to a special club that, when the chips were down, naturally bonded them.

And they were great with the patients. They would confront reeking wounds and soiled linen with a smile, while I could only grimace. They would chat to the speechless and laugh with the loveless as if it was some sort of honour: the easiest of jobs. I was envious. I just didn't have that knack. The day Shula had told me I had failed to see Mr Riley's humanity, only his body, I had been stung. But she was right. I had only seen a broken husk of a man, with a festering ulcer, who was close to death. She saw a much-loved husband and father, who'd worked all his life and now simply needed a bit of care, which she was happy to provide.

In time, I got to understand a little better. Things hit me. Like the kindness of one family, grandchildren and all, who turned up every Sunday to talk to their 'nan', even though she had been comatose for weeks, or the doggedness of a be-suited man who brought his stricken father a newspaper first thing every morning, despite his old man's loss of sight and mind. Or I'd notice Mrs Riley's love for her palsied husband, or the simple, good-heartedness of the nurses, so patient with even the most hellish and curmudgeonly souls.

I had a particular soft spot for Gillian. She was the only patient who insisted on being called by her first name, a bit unusual back then. Gillian was very sick. She had emphysema, and often needed oxygen to ease her wheezy, phlegm-clogged chest. But she was full of life, with a lucid mind and brilliant blue eyes.

'Come for a chat, young man,' she'd say, as I walked past her bed. 'Come and make my day.' She was a terrible flirt and it was hard to resist. Her stories were always worth a listen, if occasionally broken up with dreadful hawking noises to clear her throat.

On Gillian's bedside table was a sepia photo of her about to plunge into the sea. The photo showed off her evident athleticism back in the 1920s, even in her dowdy swimwear.

'That was just before my big swim,' explained Gillian, seeing me eye the photo. 'I was still in my twenties. Oh, what a time.' She smiled sadly. 'The nurses claim I swam the Channel. I didn't, actually. Got three miles from Calais and the tide was all wrong.' She shook her head. 'Never did try again. But, oh, what a memory.' She winked at me. 'I was always a bit of a wild one, you know. I fell in love with an American swimmer, who was obsessed with cold water. We used to swim at all times of the year. Brighton in December. Brrr.' She shivered at the thought. 'But, oh, what a kick to the system. You should try it, Jimmy.'

Gillian stressed the many benefits of plunging into freezing water. She told me it lowered the blood pressure, reduced cholesterol and boosted the immune system. 'And, young man, after you've thawed out,' she moved closer to me, her face all lit up, 'it makes you terribly randy.' I'm sure I blushed, receiving libido advice from this hot-wired octogenarian. 'So take an icy plunge, Jimmy, then see your girlfriend. Hah!!'

Gillian was visited by no one. She told me she'd lived life on her terms. She'd been close to marrying once, but decided against it. She'd travelled a bit, scraped a living from secretarial work, and kept swimming until last year. She had no regrets about being so sick and alone. She'd smoked too much, which had destroyed her lungs, but she saw this as a consequence rather than a punishment. Like so many of her generation, she accepted her lot. She felt she'd lived a good and lucky life.

On my final day at the hospital the nurses organised a little farewell party. Shula baked a cake, with an icing sculpture of me in a nurse's uniform, which caused much hilarity. I was grateful to all of them: that ward had taught me more about human nature than any number of years at school. And perhaps for the first time in my young life, I felt truly proud. But when Shula asked me if I might ever work in a hospital again, I told her: 'No way!'

That final afternoon Gillian had a particularly bad wheezing fit. She was fed oxygen through a mask for a while and rallied slightly. Later, I found her propped up on a sea of pillows, her hair a rook's nest of silver. Her breathing was weak, governed by its own jittery rhythms, and she looked depressed.

It was difficult for me to know how to say goodbye. I sat by her for a while and held her hand. She was completely washed out, all energy sated, and I felt horrible leaving her like that. On a whim I picked up the photo of Gillian in her swimming heyday and held it up to her face. It took a while for her to focus, and then, there it was, just briefly, a smile pricked her lips, and her blue eyes shone. Something deep down inside, a spark of former glory, rushed over her like a moment of grace.

With her hand Gillian gestured for me to move closer. 'Come back,' she whispered, smiled, and then closed her eyes. I went back three weeks later, but Gillian was already dead. That night I had a cold bath in her honour. Incredibly, twenty years later I was heading back to the wards – this time in uniform.

After my first day at nursing school and the induction by the Beards, I met up with Jake for our monthly game of snooker.

'We all had to confess today why we became nurses,' I told Jake, as we chalked our cues. I explained how the rest of the class – Chips, Vicky, Jana and co – had all provided poignant and compelling reasons.

'Oh yeah,' he replied. 'And what's your reason, Jimmy?'

'You remember that summer we went to Mexico?'

'What about it? That was years ago,' Jake said, potting two balls with one shot.

'Well, I think it's what made me want to nurse.'

One distant summer, Jake and I had volunteered to work with street children in Mexico. There had been a group of six of us – all Brits. We arrived in the swirling heart of Mexico City pale, eager and starry eyed. The first day we had taken the street kids – some as a young as eight years old – to Mexico's version of Alton Towers: a special annual treat for them. Each of us was given four children to look after. We mucked around on helter-skelters, ghost trains, water slides, and then all met up for a final roll call. To my horror, I realised one of my charges, Alberto, a lad of only ten, was gone.

'Oh, not Alberto again,' said Diego, one of the charity's Mexican staff. 'Don't worry about him, hombre. He always runs off right at the end.'

'But where did he go?' I asked. 'He's only ten. We've got to find him!'

'He'll be fine, we'll probably catch up with him later in the week.'

'But he's only ten!' I repeated. I thought back to myself at that age. I had been terrified of sleeping in the dark, let alone sleeping on the street.

'They are street kids, Jimmy,' said Diego, calmly rubbing his moustache. 'The clue is in the name. The street is Alberto's home, he's more streetwise than both of us put together. It's sad he's living rough, but that's how it is.'

I still insisted on us conducting a quick search, which as Diego expected, proved fruitless.

'You need to wise up, Jimmy,' said Diego, after we'd trawled the area. 'This is a whole new world for you.'

And it was. Many of the children at the charity's shelter had suffered physical and sexual abuse, several were HIV positive, others were addicted to drugs, booze or sniffing glue, paint or petrol. The charity's staff maintained links with the families when they could, but many of the children were utterly on their own. What really astonished me was the pull of the street, especially when street kids were viewed by many in the city as thieves and hoodlums, little better than vermin. Even though the charity had compassionate staff and decent facilities – dorms, classrooms, a health clinic, a basketball pitch – many of the children still preferred to sleep rough. The street gave them a sense of solidarity, of pride. It was a place where they were free – a place they could call home.

At the end of the month all six volunteers had been inspired by the plight of the children, and, with the naivety of youth, swore we would be back. Of course, none of us kept our promise, except one: a dynamic Scottish girl called Kay. She not only returned to Mexico, but stayed, working as a translator and trying to do her bit for street kids. Whenever I got email updates from her, it always got me thinking.

'I still think about Mexico, too,' admitted Jake, as he continued to shoot balls into pockets. 'But it wouldn't make me want to become a nurse.'

'It's not the only reason,' I said. 'But it was one of the best months of my life. And so were the weeks I volunteered at that hospital as a teenager.'

'I thought you hated that?'

'So did I!' I laughed. 'But when I look back, those two months stand out. I was actually helping people. All my other jobs were just mucking about to earn money. Now I'm older I want to do something useful again.'

'You do realise, Jimmy,' said Jake, finally missing a shot, 'that Bill and I don't have perfect jobs either. I often think I'm just treading water.' He shrugged. 'Teaching foreigners English is hardly rocket science. I'm not even challenging myself by teaching kids – just adults, all eager to learn.'

'But you're a great teacher,' I insisted. 'And Bill enjoys his work, or at least his salary. And his main concern has always been providing for his family.'

My own eight-year-old daughter, nicknamed Poppin, had moved overseas recently. I had split with her mother some time ago. She had always been Poppin's centre of gravity, her home star. I had simply been a meteor with visitation rights, whizzing into her life and out again, a whirl of irresponsible love. My ex was now happily remarried and my daughter was in a grounded and secure environment. This comforted me, but her absence hurt like hell at times.

Before Poppin left I had been seeing her weekly but now she was miles away across the Atlantic. I still wrote and spoke to her regularly but only saw her once a year. Her departure no doubt acted as a further catalyst for my move into nursing.

'Mate, it's obvious, all your midlife crises have come at once,' said Jake, setting up the balls for a fresh game. 'That's why you're nursing.'

'And don't try to defend me.' Jake grinned. 'I'm a dedicated teacher now, but I wasn't at the beginning. I just used it as a way to meet girls.'

'There's something magnificent about your shallowness, Jake.'

To be fair, Jake, even back at school, had always been a wow with the girls. I could never understand this because he used to have the most diabolically uncool taste in music. While the rest of us were air-guitaring to the Clash and the Ramones, he hummed along to Andrew Lloyd Webber. What teenage girl in her right mind would want her precious first kiss accompanied to 'Magical Mr Mistoffelees'? Well, lots of them. Jake made no effort to be hip, and as a consequence had queues of hormonal damsels swooning at his moccasined feet. While I, his oh-so-trendy best mate would stew in monkish frustration listening to Elvis Costello wail about thwarted love, revolution and spots.

Jake had continued to land on his feet throughout life. He was now a respected teacher and engaged to one of his ex-students, a lovely Spanish lawyer called Anna, to whom he was devoted.

'So what does Jess think about your nursing?' Jake asked. 'You don't want to lose her, Jimmy. She's far too good for you.'

Ah, yes, Jess, my effervescent girlfriend, who was indeed far too good for me. Jess and I had got together a while before I began the degree. She was supportive of my nursing but fearful that the long hours would reduce my stamina. She could happily party until the early hours – she was a few years younger than me – while I, it soon became clear, was ready to crash long before midnight with a mug of cocoa and a medical text book.

Jess was also a fan of extreme sports. She was training for the Marathon des Sables, a punishing week-long race across the Sahara Desert, during which she would carry all her own kit in mercury-busting heat. To train for this appalling ordeal I would accompany her on fifty-mile yomps and vigorous cycle rides at the weekends. She would come back from these fired up and ready for more, while I would be frazzled and half dead.

I never really understood Jess's work. She was some sort of IT whizz, and was often away travelling. It amused me that she worked in a profession dominated by men, and I was now in one surrounded by women. I teased her for being a fat-cat bonus chaser, while she wrote me off as a technophobic old geezer. In many ways it was a great relationship and Jess was a lovely and loving presence in my life. But at times it was hard keeping up with her near-Olympian levels of energy. A question mark hovered over our future together.

'Hang on to Jess, mate, she's a sweetheart,' Jake reinforced. He scraped fresh chalk on his cue and surveyed the baize. 'Is she cool with the nursing?'

'She's fine with it so far,' I replied.

'To be honest, mate,' Jake said, 'when I first heard you wanted to nurse I thought you were a complete pussy.' He smashed the cue ball down the table. 'But, hey, I suppose what you're doing takes balls, too.'

'Thanks, Jake,' I said, as I pondered on the biological impossibility of his statement. 'That makes me feel much better.'

Chapter 3

TOO COOL FOR SCHOOL

Back at college some strong friendships were already being forged. The two Muslim girls Hadia and Shima, both away from home for the first time, were inseparable. Sheena, Coco and Ola formed another tentative posse and Mayla, always a law unto herself, flitted between us all – at least when she could tear herself away from the latest Mills and Boon bodice ripper. Esme, a sullen teenager from Hounslow, only appeared sporadically and never mingled with the rest of us, and a girl called Penny never showed up at all.

Chips – the Shamrock snapper, Jana – the Bermudan brainbox, Vicky – an earthy Essex girl, and I – a son of the shires, formed another multi-culti quartet. We were an incongruous bunch in age, race and upbringing, but somehow clicked.

We teased each other non-stop. Jana, for her addiction to internet dating sites; Vicky, for her grungy dress sense and constant nicotine fixes; Chips, for being hopelessly forgetful and having a rakish taste in hats; and me, for my inability to master predictive text and my fogeyish rants about the modern world, reality TV and 'too many bloody Starbucks'.

Despite the formation of little cliques, we all rubbed along well as a group, too, except for Esme, who clearly wanted nothing to do with any of us, and Penny, who remained invisible.

The lessons with the Beards were the best for group bonding, and we would all come away on a high after learning skills that might potentially save a life.

Much of our time with the Beards was spent taking each others' pulses, temperatures, respirations and blood pressures. These skills are known as 'basic observations' or 'the obs' and are essential for a student nurse to master before being unleashed on the wards.

Several students, such as Vicky and Hadia, already knew how to do 'the obs' having recently volunteered in a hospital. They knew that an adult pulse beats around 60 to 80 times a minute – while a newborn baby's can beat up to 180 times ('Same as mine whenever I see Johnny Depp,' cooed Jana). They knew we breathe on average 12 to 20 times a minute (a baby up to 50 times) and that the average human temperature is between 36 to 37 degrees Celsius (96.8 to 98.6 degrees Fahrenheit for those of you who, like my mum, still have mercury thermometers).

In comparison, I was clueless. In fact, the first time I took Vicky's pulse I put my thumb on her wrist, instead of my finger.

'Never use a thumb to take a pulse, Jimmy,' urged Robbie, drawing my hand away. 'Your thumb has its own pulse, so you might feel that rather than your patient's. Always use your fingers.'

But taking a pulse was child's play compared to reading a blood pressure (or BP). Indeed, a BP reading is every trainee nurse's nightmare – but essential to master.

'Blood pressure is a key indicator of health,' stressed Rob. 'Pain, fear, anxiety and being an unhealthy geezer like me with clogged arteries,' he rubbed his belly for effect, 'tends to cause high blood pressure.'

'While being fighting fit like yours truly,' said Robbie (I hope this was a joke as he was just as portly as Rob) 'usually gives you low BP. As does dehydration, severe infection, loss of blood or a rise in temperature.'

'A rise in temperature causes low blood pressure,' said Jana. 'That doesn't make sense, does it?

Robbie explained that having a high temperature tends to cause sweating. This in turn widens the blood vessels, thus easing the pressure on them. He also stressed BP readings were complex and there were always exceptions to rules, such as a physically fit person having high blood pressure due to a heavy cholesterol diet.

This all made sense, but now came the hard part – taking the bloody readings. This involves a machine called a sphygmomanometer (one of those nice, catchy medical words), and a stethoscope. The idea is to work out both the systolic* pressure (when the blood pumped from the heart is at maximum pressure against the arteries), compared to the diastolic pressure (when the heart is resting, and the blood pressure on the arteries is at its weakest).

So far, so good. But to measure these pressures you need to juggle skills like one of those multi-armed Hindu goddesses. One: wrap a cuff around the patient's upper arm. Two: explain what you are doing. Three: pump up the cuff. Four: gradually deflate it. Five: Use a stethoscope to listen to the changes in the pulse of the brachial artery.

Ah, the brachial artery! Compared to the radial pulse on the wrist, finding the brachial pulse on the upper arm is like trying to locate the lost city of Shangri-La. Fumbling around with my fingers I couldn't find Chips's brachial pulse, I couldn't find Sheena's, I couldn't find Rob's – I couldn't even find my own. Finally, I came up trumps with Vicky, who had a brachial pulse like a spurting geyser.

---

*When you hear doctors or paramedics shouting 'asystole!' in hospital soaps (*ER* staff use the word a lot) it means some unfortunate patient's heart shows no activity at all – or rather some hapless actor is unlikely to get any more lines.

Then, putting the stethoscope's dial on Vicky's arm, I slowly released the pressure from the cuff and watched the gauge on the sphygmomanometer (or sphyg, to use its less fearsome nickname). While doing this I listened through the stethoscope's ear pieces to Vicky's brachial pulse, which was now soft as tiptoes. Finally, I noted the two readings of when I heard her pulse start and stop – this being her blood pressure.

'Bad news, Vicky,' I told her. 'You've got a blood pressure higher than Ozzy Osbourne. Or maybe you're pregnant!'

'I've actually got very low BP, Jimmy,' said Vicky. 'I think it's more likely you've made a complete cock-up with the reading.'

At first I thought it would be easier to write Sanskrit or master the bassoon than to take an accurate blood pressure reading. It seemed extraordinarily hard. But Jana, Vicky, Chips and I practised obsessively on each other, and slowly we began to crack it. Soon it gave us all great pleasure to shout out 'BP fine, 120 over 80' or 'BP high, 163 over 96'★ with the confidence of seasoned paramedics.

Whether in class, taking each others' pulses or lunching in the hospital canteen, our little group had really started to pull together – except for Esme.

Esme still kept her distance. We tried to be friendly, blend her into conversations, but she was having none of it. The missing Penny may have been more sanguine, but we never found out. Mr Temple told us one morning that Penny had quit. Well, quit seems a bit strong; she hadn't ever joined us.

In truth, Esme didn't look as though she was going to stick it out either. She seemed the least likely nurse imaginable. She spent most of the classes scowling, blowing bubble gum and furtively listening to her iPod. At the end of each lesson she would sigh: 'God, that was borrrr-ing.'

★Blood pressure is measured in millimetres of mercury (mmHG).

I found Esme's attitude hard to fathom. Having spent much of my school days larking about, I was now at an age when I really wanted to learn. Other mature students such as Chips and Sheena shared my excitement. Sheena, the grandmother of the group, told Esme she needed to buck up her ideas.

'You are letting us all down, young lady,' Sheena, ever straight talking, told her one lunchtime. 'You never smile. You never show any interest. If you were nursing me I would be terrified. You will be on the wards soon. Start shaping up.'

To be fair to Esme, while some lectures were inspiring, others were crushingly dull. I found those focusing on communication skills especially trying. The buzz word always seemed to be 'empathy' – or 'putting yourself in somebody else's boots', as the Beards put it.

Of course, I realised showing empathy was vital for a nurse, but I had a problem with having it drummed into me on an almost hourly basis. 'Don't forget empathy! Be empathetic! Empathise!' To my mind, empathy is not a quality that can be forced on anyone. Like a beautiful singing voice or a good eye for a ball, both of which sadly elude me, you need to have a natural reservoir of it in the first place for it to truly develop. You either have a gift for it, or you don't. And if not, empathy is more likely to be nurtured by experience rather than in class.

Many of the group had empathy flowing through their veins. Others possessed a healthy syringeful, and a few stragglers like me had a small enough dose to get by. But Esme seemed so bereft of empathy that, bar a visit to the Wizard of Oz, nothing would help.

In fact, Esme not only lacked empathy, but wanted to actively blow a raspberry at it. She seemed thoroughly pissed off with the world. When asked by one lecturer to take somebody's temperature she simply told them: 'I can't be bothered.' Even Mr Temple did not faze her. When he told her she needed to show more humility, Esme's reply was: 'Whatever!' When Mr Temple told her to leave the class, she shrugged and walked out. Sheena and Chips tried to talk to her, but she refused to engage.

Predictably, Esme (and the elusive Penny) were the first to quit the course. Esme lasted about six weeks, leaving shortly before we were to start our first placements in the hospital. In some ways, I was glad she never reached the wards. Her boot-faced attitude would hardly fill her patients' hearts with cheer. I'm sure she's got a great future in law, or poker, or nihilistic philosophy – just not nursing.

But perhaps I was guilty of showing Esme a complete lack of empathy myself. Maybe she was just going through a hard time, had issues none of us could understand. But by not talking with any of us, it was impossible for us to find out. It was a shame to lose two of our group so early, but it was certainly clear that in the case of Esme she was on the wrong course at the wrong time.

As Sheena said: 'Jimmy, that young lady was just too cool for school.'

Or as the ever-empathetic Mr Temple put it: 'Two down, ten to go.'

Chapter 4

LAST MAN STANDING

The last day at school before heading to the wards we spent learning Cardio Pulmonary Resuscitation (or CPR). I'd been looking forward to this one.

In its most basic terms, CPR is a means to keep the blood flowing around the body in the absence of a pulse. It's a fundamental skill. And yet, how many of us know how to do it? How many times have we walked past a scene where a person is collapsed and we have simply looked on, unable to lift a finger? And we are not the only ones: often there is a cast of frozen observers. Of course, you sometimes hear those splendid words: 'Let me through, I'm a doctor/nurse/first aider'. But this is not often the case. Usually nobody knows what the hell is going on until an ambulance turns up, by which stage it's often too late.

I certainly know I've been guilty of this. Several years ago I stumbled upon a scene – an elderly woman had collapsed in a park, her shopping scattered everywhere. She had landed hard, and a damson-coloured bruise already dominated her face. She was also bleeding profusely from a cut above her eyebrow. The poor woman looked as crumpled as if she'd been dropped from the sky. I'd asked someone in the crowd if an ambulance had already been called. It had. Oh good! Great news! But now my potential use was at an end. I simply stood, along with lots of other concerned but useless souls, waiting for the paramedics to work their magic. It was terrible being so powerless.

One time this powerlessness spread closer to home. The previous summer my septuagenarian cousin had collapsed at a party. The assembled guests had gathered around his prostrate body, unsure what to do. It was truly grim, seeing your favourite cousin on the floor, ashen faced and blue lipped. His walking stick had fallen across him like the rifle of a stricken soldier. The assembled crowd looked down at him with great compassion, but nobody had a clue what to do.

In a panic, I finally tracked down a doctor among the party guests – a young, sharply dressed brunette – who took instant control of the situation. She carefully put a cushion under my cousin's legs, and another one under his head, and soon the blood supply returned to his vital organs. It was so simple. My cousin then rallied and, looking up at the angelic young doctor, said: 'Thank God, I've gone to heaven.'

My cousin was rushed to hospital, underwent endless tests, and was released later in the evening. He was advised not to eat anything heavy or drink alcohol. With typical panache he wolfed several forkfuls of chicken chow mein washed down with a glass of Rioja, and woke up the next morning right as rain. Despite the happy ending, seeing someone I loved in this state made me realise the importance of first aid, and how few of us out there know even the basics.

Personally, I think all school pupils should have compulsory first aid lessons. First aid teaches biology, responsibility and, yes, empathy, all in one. Given my time again I'd much rather have learnt how to bring someone back to life than sweat over long division or the conjugation of French verbs.

The good news was that our CPR lesson would be taught by the Beards. The bad news was that Mr Temple was helping them out. We were split into two groups, one with Robbie and Rob and one with Mr Temple. I was peeled off into Mr Temple's team. Oh joy! I could see Chips, Hadia, Shima, Jana and Vicky all felt the same way.

Mr Temple began by asking us some questions. First up: How long should it take an ambulance to reach somebody in an emergency?

'Twenty minutes,' said Chips, confidently.

Mr Temple grimaced and nodded his head.

'Fifteen minutes,' guessed Vicky.

'No, no, no!' Mr Temple snorted. 'Good God! You call fifteen minutes urgent. I'd be as dead as Julius Caesar by then. It's eight minutes. Eight! OK!'

We all mumbled 'yes', as solemnly as a church congregation. His next question was: What are the success rates of reviving someone by CPR?

'Fifty-fifty,' said Hadia. Mr Temple slapped his forehead in despair.

'One in three,' Sheena suggested.

'No, no, no!' he groaned. 'Don't any of you read? It's only between 5 and 10 per cent.'

Mr Temple added that CPR success depended on how quickly it was given after someone's heart had stopped. Any time beyond ten minutes, he stressed, with rather too much relish, and 'not even Lazarus could be resuscitated'.

My upbeat mood was rapidly fading.

Now we got down to the nitty-gritty – what to do if we came across a collapsed body. Mr Temple walked to a white board and wrote in big, very neat letters the acronym: AAAABC, telling us this was all we needed to know.

Mr Temple explained that the first A stood for Approach – to make sure the area around the body was safe ('No live wires or toxic spillages or things to trip over'), and the second A for Assess – to check whether the patient is conscious. He ordered me to lie down on the floor.

'Right,' said Mr Temple. 'How am I going to check if Jimmy is conscious?'

'Watch him' said Jana, tentatively. 'See if he's moving.'

'Genius!' Mr Temple got down on his knees and crouched over me. 'But I'm also going to talk to him. Ask him to open his eyes. Gently shake his shoulders.'

'Can you hear me?' Mr Temple asked, shaking my shoulders, but not gently at all. In fact, he was as frantic as Kate Winslet trying to revive Leonardo DiCaprio at the end of *Titanic*. I began to feel a bit nauseous. 'Can you hear me, Jimmy?'

'Yes,' I whispered.

'You're supposed to be unconscious, man! Shut up and pretend to be dead.'

We next learnt that the third A stands for Airway. Mr Temple put a hand on my forehead and tilted back my head, letting my mouth fall open to check it wasn't blocked ('No obstruction there, thank God') and the fourth A for Assistance – meaning to shout for help ('good and loud!').

'Help! Help!' screamed Mr Temple, again doing a passable impression of Kate Winslet, only slightly more excitable. The Beards looked across at us with growing concern. Their group was having a distinctly more relaxed session on the other side of the room.

Chips rushed over to help, but was forcefully rejected by Mr Temple. 'Imagine I'm in the hills, man. There is no help available. Just me. Me and some mountain goats. Got it!' Chips backed off. I had a disturbing image of Mr Temple halfway up the Matterhorn with goat bells chiming in the background. Julie Andrews was nowhere in sight.

Next up was the letter B, which we were told stood for Breathing. Mr Temple moved his ear close to my mouth, looking down over my body to see if I was drawing breath.

'Listen and look for breath,' said Mr Temple. 'And feel for breath against your ear.' He moved his ear a little bit closer to my face. I held my breath and stayed still as a statue.

After ten seconds Mr Temple surfaced. He explained that if someone was still breathing at this stage they should be put into the recovery position. To demonstrate he deftly manipulated me on to my side, so my mouth faced downwards. This, he told us, would keep my airway clear and would mean I was safe if I vomited or choked.

But if I wasn't breathing, Mr Temple said, man-handling me on to my back again, then we have to check for C.

'C for Circulation, people,' he shouted. 'To check it we need to find the carotid artery. This part isn't essential but useful if you can do it – and as a nurse you should be able to!'

He pointed at Hadia, and told her to pinpoint my carotid artery. Hadia, clearly nervous, knelt down by my side and put her finger tentatively to the side of my Adam's apple.

'Apply a bit of pressure, dear,' urged Mr Temple. 'You look as if you're defusing a bomb.'

'I can feel his pulse,' said Hadia, delighted.

'No, you can't,' corrected Mr Temple. 'Jimmy's heart has stopped, remember.' With this he ushered Hadia away without praise, announcing: 'It's time for compressions.'

Mr Temple overlapped his hands, and, palms face down, placed them on the centre of my chest.

'So now,' he stated loudly. 'I give thirty compressions!'

'No way!' I thought, cricking my neck up.

'Don't look so nervous, Jimmy,' said Mr Temple, smiling grimly. 'I'll use another volunteer, instead.'

The rest of the group simultaneously took a couple of steps back. Mr Temple glared at them. His pallid face glowered with whole decades' worth of anger, disappointment and bile.

'Don't worry, I'm not using any of you! I'm using George!' Mr Temple stood up and walked over to a bed with a plastic dummy lying on top of it. That must be George, I realised, the poor fellow. Mr Temple grabbed the well-toned dummy and placed him on the floor, kneeling over him. He put his palms on the middle of George's chest, just below the rib cage and, keeping his arms straight, began to press down.

'How many times do I have to do this?' he said, pumping up and down. Was it me, or did George look decidedly anxious?

'Thirty,' said Vicky.

'Bravo! A right answer for a change!' Mr Temple was soon beginning to run out of steam, his face reddening. 'How fast do I give the compressions?' There was a long pause – just the sound of George's body clicking up and down.

'At a rate of 100 a minute,' gasped Mr Temple. 'You should know this.' He told us 100 times a minute was the exact speed of the song 'Nellie the Elephant', and we could sing it as we did our compressions as a way to remember.

Incredibly, Mr Temple then started to sing: 'Nellie the elephant packed her truck.' He kept the words in exact time to the compressions. 'And said goodbye to the cir-cus! Off she went with a trumpety trump. Trump, trump, *trump*!'

I couldn't believe my eyes, let alone my ears. This was a vision that would remain with me for the rest of my days, however hard I tried to eradicate it. Mr Temple trying to revive an enlarged Action Man while singing about an elephant on its way to Mandalay. Trump, trump, *trump*! By the time he had completed his compressions and spirited rendition of 'Nellie the Elephant' I thought Mr Temple might need CPR himself, for he had turned a peculiar shade of purple.

After he had regained his breath, Mr Temple told us that the Queen song, 'Another One Bites the Dust', was also a good one to work out the speed of compressions, but could be seen as being a little disrespectful, especially if the CPR didn't work.

Mr Temple finished up by explaining that once the thirty compressions were over, two rescue breaths were needed. He put his palm over George's forehead and tilted back his head, before lowering himself to give a couple of rescue breaths – or what used to be called 'kisses of life'.

'Phew,' said Vicky, watching the dummy's plastic ribcage inflate. 'I'm so happy I'm not George.'

After this Mr Temple gamely continued to try to resuscitate George, explaining that we should continue to do thirty compressions and two rescue breaths until help arrives or until we 'conk out'.

Only once Mr Temple had stopped did Hadia raise her hand.

'Sorry, sir,' she said, peering out from her black headdress. 'But what was all that stuff about elephants?'

In retrospect, I'm glad it was Mr Temple who taught us that day. He made us repeat AAAABC on George and on each other, until we were completely fed up. If any of us forgot Assess or Airway, or performed one of the tasks incorrectly, he would berate us without mercy.

'That's not a compression, Shima, you wouldn't revive a dormouse with that!'

'He's breathing, Chips. No point resuscitating someone who's already breathing!'

'Calm down, Vicky, you could blow up an air balloon with that sort of kiss – I don't want George to explode.'

We did not stop until every one of us could perform CPR pitch perfect. We were hassled and humiliated, and went on half an hour longer than the other group. But not one of us would ever forget what to do the next time we saw a collapsed body. Mr Temple may have been a bit of a bully, a bit scary and pedantic, but CPR was the subject he was born to teach. I remember every word of the lesson even now, and for that I will always be grateful.

Despite our grumbling at Mr Temple's grilling we were all pumped up as we headed out for lunch. It was a warm day and we decided to grab a sandwich and sit in a small communal garden opposite the hospital. Mayla, who had missed the CPR session, was basking on a bench, her nose in a Mills and Boon romance called *The Duchess of Destiny*. We sat ourselves around her.

Mayla told us she was missing her boyfriend Chad, a US marine, who was posted in Japan. She also felt nursing was not really her thing, and had decided to quit the course. Jana and Vicky tried to change her mind, but Mayla was not for turning.

'I'm love sick,' she pined, hugging her arms to her chest. 'Chad is the love of my life, my destiny. I must go to him. He has my heart.' She really had been reading far too many Mills and Boon.

As Mayla rhapsodised over her distant lover, Chips appeared. He had stayed on at school after Mr Temple's lesson to collect some books from the library. He slumped down on the grass between Vicky and Jana. He had a piece of paper in his hand.

'I'm out, guys,' said Chips, waving the paper above his head. 'My criminal records check has just come through.' He shook his head. 'I've been kicked off for driving without insurance. I didn't have my MOT either.'

'You can appeal,' Jana told him. 'No insurance shouldn't stop you being a nurse.'

'I was caught within the last six months,' said Chips. 'That's my problem.'

This was a shock. I really liked Chips and thought he would be a good nurse – compassionate, intuitive, funny. Surely dodging his MOT and insurance, though extremely foolish, shouldn't jeopardise his character so much as to make him unfit for the wards. But I also had more selfish reasons – I didn't want to be the only male member of the group: the last man standing.

'I'll have to wait a year until starting the course again,' said Chips. 'I can't afford it. I'm sorry guys, it's been great but I'm out. Back to photography.'

'You can't leave us, Chips,' Vicky implored, stubbing out her cigarette. 'Without you, Jimmy will be overwhelmed by oestrogen.'

'He should be so lucky,' said Jana, putting her arm round Chips.

Chips had been due to work in the same children's ward as Vicky, Ola and me on our first placement. We had visited the ward the day before, enjoyed meeting the staff, and were all looking forward to starting there on Monday.

What a blow for Chips. Mayla had always seemed a bit half-hearted about nursing but Chips had been the most fired up of all of us. It seemed such a shame he was leaving, a waste of potential. We all exchanged contact details and Chips told us about a photography exhibition he was putting on in a few weeks' time. We all agreed to meet then.

Penny, Esme, Mayla and Chips: even before we had reached the wards, a quarter of our group were out. But this was to be just the start. Incredibly, within a couple of months only half of us would remain. Indeed, by the end of the first year there would be very few of us left. The reasons for departure varied – disillusion, aversion to bodily fluids, exam failure, dwindling funds and family responsibility all conspired to decimate our little gang.

I had seen Mr Temple as the ultimate doom-monger – 'some of you simply will not survive!' – spouting fate like some old hag from a morality play. But he had been right about dropout rates after all. In fact, regarding our group, he had even been underestimating.

Four down, eight to go.

Chapter 5

ONTO THE WARDS

The weekend flew by and next thing I knew it was dawn on Monday – time for my first shift as a student nurse. My alarm jangled me to life. I showered, swigged some coffee, threw a few snacks into my rucksack and cycled off into the dark. Two minutes later I was back again – I'd forgotten my JIMMY FRAZIER – STUDENT NURSE identification badge and the packed lunch Jess had prepared for me.

Pedalling to the ward, which was nowhere near the nursing school, took nearly an hour. But it wasn't this that irked me, or the monsoon-like rain, or the fact I'd got up at cock crow, or even that Sheffield Wednesday had lost again at the weekend.

It was the fact there was nowhere to change into my uniform. On arrival at the ward I'd asked for the locker room. I was told that the nurses didn't have a locker room but a 'station' – a communal place where we could dump our kit, write our notes and drink our tea. I poked my head into the 'station'. It was tiny – the size of a garden shed – and already so chock-full of nurses, that many of them were standing. I asked where I could change into my uniform.

'In the staff toilet round the back,' said a girl with gingery hair, reading a computer screen. 'Hurry though, we're starting handover soon.'

'Change in a toilet!' I said.

'Yes, out the back, we're short of space. Hurry now.'

I was dumbfounded. In my imagination all hospitals had swanky locker rooms – at least they did on TV. From *Casualty* to *Scrubs* the locker room was the staff nerve centre: a place to unwind, to gossip, to escape the hubbub of the ward, and most pressingly, change into your uniform. But, oh no. We had a station – a station so full we couldn't even change in it.

Outside the toilet I bumped into Vicky. She was battling to wake up. She was so dazed it seemed she'd been hit over the head with a frying pan.

'I can't believe it's only 7 a.m.,' she groaned, combing her unruly blond hair. I noticed she had removed her crucifix earrings and all her other jewellery – a ward rule.

'So where did you change?' I asked.

'In there!' She pointed at the toilet door. 'How unhygienic is that!'

I had to agree with her. At lectures it was drummed into us never to wear our uniforms outside of the hospital. This was to cut the risk of picking up germs away from the clinical setting. Even if we dashed to the local shops at lunch break we still had to change. This made perfect sense. What didn't make sense was putting our uniforms on again in a room swarming with bacteria.

The 'dressing toilet' was clean enough, but small, dingy and airless. With MRSA running rampant through hospitals across the country, this poky thunder-box was something of a shock. To be fair, the hospital, which was well over 100 years old, was currently undergoing a radical makeover – and not a moment too soon.

As I came out from my cubicle, Ola appeared from a door opposite. As always, she looked immaculate, her swirling robes now replaced by a neatly ironed blue uniform. She had sensibly changed in the patients' bathroom, giving herself more space despite flouting the rules.

'I'm so flipping nervous,' said Ola. 'I haven't slept at all.' Vicky put her arm around her and we all scurried off to handover.

Handovers are intimidating at first. You are stuck in a jam-packed room surrounded by strangers who communicate only in nurse speak; a mix of medical jargon, patient updates and the juiciest of hospital gossip.

The purpose of a handover is for a nurse from the previous shift to tell the new shift what's been going on. As this ward was known as 'a gastro ward' (this did not extend to the food, sadly) its beds were filled with children – from newborn babies to seventeen-year-olds – suffering from any number of gut-related problems.

Vicky, Ola and I stood sardined in a corner, listening to a matronly Jamaican nurse update us. Considering she had started her shift more than twelve hours earlier, and it was her fourth night in a row, I expected her to sound like some jaded, late-night DJ, but she was very cheery. She spoke in the hard, muscular language of medicine, using words like hypertensive, analgesia and ileostomy ('for all you students, any word ending in 'stomy', means something with a hole in it!'). But she used more easily graspable language, too: 'When little Leroy in Bed Three gets anxious, read him *The Gruffalo*.'

The handover lasted twenty minutes, by which time all the nurses had been allocated roles for the day. As students, Vicky, Ola and I were all 'supernumerary'. This demoralising title basically means superfluous.

If I didn't feel superfluous yet, I did soon after meeting my mentor. All student nurses have a mentor. The word 'mentor' sounds very Zen – the enlightened teacher grooming the callow novice. It doesn't always work out like this. While some mentors are generous and eager to pass on their skills, others only become mentors to get promotion. The latter types see students as lower than cockroaches in the wheel of life. My mentor, a small, joyless woman called Cathy, set me firmly in this category.

Indeed, when I told her she was my mentor, Cathy looked me up and down and said: 'No I'm not!' With a toss of her hair, she walked away. I spoke to the ward sister, a kind but very busy woman called Isobel, who assured me that Cathy was my mentor. Next time I confronted Cathy she was her usual charming self.

'OK, OK,' she snapped. 'I'll be your bloody mentor if I have to.'

With this attitude, I sensed my path to nursing enlightenment would be a long one.

It transpired that Snappy Cathy, as I nicknamed her, had been a veterinary nurse early in her career, before shifting to humans. She kept a photo of her pet poodle on her mobile phone screen saver – the poor thing had been manicured into a canine version of Paris Hilton. Sadly, Snappy's love of hapless creatures didn't extend to students.

On the plus side, Snappy kept me on my toes. Every shift she insisted I joined her to perform routine 'obs' on all the children, whether tiny babies or teenagers. I would also help her prepare any medication. She was always meticulous over this, inspecting capsules and measuring liquids with the grace of an alchemist.

'Never mess up a child's medication,' said Snappy, holding up a syringe. 'A dose that hardly affects an adult can kill a baby in minutes. There can be no drug errors on this ward.'

It was good advice. In our final year as trainee nurses we had to take a drug calculation exam and pass it 100 per cent. Even 99 per cent didn't cut it. And quite rightly: that 1 per cent error might mean a dead child. Maths was not my strong point – I would need to really up my game. I didn't want to become known as Nurse Herod.

At the end of the first week I felt shattered. I had learnt a lot but my mentor's blatant hostility wasn't exactly boosting my confidence. The babies on the ward didn't take a shine to me, either. Much like Snappy, they pulled Edvard Munch–like screams every time I so much as looked at them. I had to concede Vicky and Ola, from what little I had seen of them, appeared to be much more naturally gifted nurses.

So when I accompanied Ola to the bus stop after our Friday shift I was surprised to hear she was struggling, too.

'Is it your mentor?' I asked.

'No, she's lovely,' said Ola, jumping on her bus. 'I'm just not sure I'm cut out for this. It's just so hard being around sick kids.' She waved at me as her bus pulled away. 'I'll talk to you next week, Jimmy.'

The following week started better for Ola. She told me she had pulled herself together over the weekend and now felt stronger. It turned out better for me, too. Snappy took some annual leave (the Alps, I believe – all that glacial air would suit her) and I was temporarily taken under the wing of an angelic senior staff nurse called Jenny.

Angelic is an overused word when it comes to nurses. Some are verging on demonic. They drink, smoke and swear like sailors. This doesn't make them bad nurses, though, as long as they act compassionately and professionally on the wards.

Vicky, Jana and I all certainly drank, swore (like polite sailors) and smoked (I passively inhaled enough of their cigarettes to be an honorary smoker). But Jenny was different. I'm sure she was vice free. She radiated goodness in the same way Mr Temple radiated spleen. Her smile could melt the hardest of hearts, and she saw the best in everyone – even Snappy. ('I think it's sweet she has her poodle on her phone'). But Jenny was no pushover. When Ola arrived late for a shift, she was taken aside. Ola was never late again. Jenny did not have to bully us, she was someone you simply didn't want to let down.

Having Jenny as a stand-in mentor made me feel much more at home on the ward, and I became more confident with the patients. Rather than buzzing around doing 'obs' on everyone, Jenny advised me to focus on one or two patients and really get to know them.

The first patient I focused on was Julius, a rangy, fourteen-year-old Brazilian boy with Crohn's disease, which had caused a serious inflammation in his intestines. A month before he had been his class joker, captain of the local basketball team and had a golden future ahead of him. Now he was bed-bound, emotionally shell-shocked and feeding through a tube.

Julius was unlucky on two counts. Crohn's disease tends to affect white Europeans and Julius was a rare exception. He was also younger than the usual Crohn's patients, as it tends to strike people in their twenties or late teens. And, perhaps most harshly, Julius had a really bad case of the disease. His ileum, the longest part of his lower intestine, was not only inflamed but ulcerated. He was in a lot of pain.

To add salt to his wounds, Julius had just come down with MRSA. Now he was in an isolated cubicle where the medical team always had to wear gloves and aprons.

Poor Julius. A photo by his bed showed a beaming, happy-go-lucky child, holding a basketball. But the new Julius seemed so mute, so broken. It was easy to understand why. One minute he had been larking around with his schoolmates and flirting with girls, next he was imprisoned in a cell smelling of disinfectant, tended by gloved strangers and, to use his words: 'dossing about in bed and pissing in a bag'.

Visiting Julius's room was like attending a death scene. His mother slumped by her son's side, saying tearful prayers. There was a photo of her by Julius's bed, a glamorous woman with bright lipstick – with her life still intact before her son's illness.

In many ways I found Julius's mental state more of a worry than his physical decline. The nurses on the ward were very skilled at cheering the sick, but none made any sort of break-through with Julius. It was hard to find any trace of the buoyant, smiling child in the photo. Even Jenny couldn't work her magic.

Julius's father, a tall, intense man, approached his son's fate in a different way. He refused to accept it. He brought in Julius's sports trophies and a poster of Beyoncé dancing in a mini-skirt. He told Julius that the doctors would work something out. He proudly recounted his son's sporting triumphs to the nurses: 'with a basketball my boy's a genius . . . ' I wondered if he realised his son might never shoot hoops again. But then I would see him alone outside Julius's room, his head in his hands, his hope as receded as his hairline. Clearly Julius's father did understand, but, at least in company, wanted to stay strong. I admired him for that.

As a student nurse I had more time than the staff nurses to talk to Julius. I tried striking up conversations but had no luck. It wasn't surprising. He was a young, cool sporting hero and I was a middle-aged student, who hadn't shot a hoop in years. But I didn't take it personally. In Julius's current state, it seemed no one could cheer him up, not even Beyoncé, all legs and teeth, beaming out from the opposite wall.

'Just give Julius time,' said Jenny. 'He's in a period of mourn-ing. He's yet to grasp he's no longer the school heart-throb. He'll come round. Trust me.'

As Julius often wanted to be alone, I spent time with another patient, Anouka, a recently admitted Tanzanian girl, with duo-denal pains and chronic diarrhoea. The doctors were unsure of the exact nature of her illness and were busily looking into it. On top of this, the smiley, frizzy-haired Anouka, just sixteen years old, was HIV positive.

Her parents, a dignified, well-dressed couple, who rarely left her bedside, told us that Anouka had gone through a wild phase last year. They were strong Baptists, and their daughter had rebelled. Over the summer she had run off for a few weeks and stayed with a cousin in Birmingham. The cousin was 'a bad seed, a terrible influence'. While staying with her, Anouka had unprotected sex at a couple of parties and had become infected.

'Perhaps we were too strict,' Anouka's father told me one morning in the hospital garden. 'We have daily prayers. Anouka's sisters all respect this. But she was always the rebel.' He smiled. 'She is a good girl really and, praise God, now we have her back.'

It was true: Anouka did seem back in the family fold. Her parents read her Bible excerpts, and when some of her siblings turned up, they would form a semicircle around her bed, link hands, and pray for her. I'm not religious, but it was a rather beautiful sight.

Anouka told me her side of the story while I did her 'obs' one morning. She said she had felt suffocated by the Christian rituals of her father, and wanted to break free. She admitted she hero-worshipped the 'bad seed' cousin who led her astray, but now realised that by running from her family she had behaved 'like a mad cow'.

Anouka came across as good hearted and full of remorse. She told me she loved her family and didn't want to hurt them any more. She was now determined to become a teacher. At times, Anouka seemed streetwise way beyond her years and then she'd say something like: 'I'm such a hopeless spaz,' and you realised she was still just a schoolgirl.

To have rebelled so briefly with such devastating results was a cruel fate for someone so young. For all her pluck, in one of her darker hours Anouka confided: 'How can I believe in a God who has done all this to me?'

Anouka found out about her new illness during my last week on the ward – Hodgkin's lymphoma, a cancer originating from the white blood cells. After some initial tears, Anouka's huge, brave smile was back in place. 'Complete bummer, Jimmy.

Don't worry though, I'll be all right. I'll beat it. I'm gonna be a teacher, remember.'

Once it was known she had Hodgkin's, Anouka was soon ferried off to another hospital. Hodgkin's does have high survival rates but Anouka's HIV would have weakened her immune system. Still, it was clear that despite all life had thrown at her so far, this was a girl who looked to the future.

'What grim luck,' I remember saying to Vicky on the day Anouka heard about her cancer. 'Isolated from other kids, plugged into drips and a question mark over her future. How does she keep her pecker up? It's incredible.'

Vicky beckoned me to follow her into Anouka's cubicle. She looked down fondly at the sleeping teenager. 'Doesn't matter how old you are, Jimmy,' said Vicky, sweeping some stray hairs away from Anouka's face. 'Some people are destroyed by unfairness – others aren't.'

Simple words, but they have stuck with me to this day.

Although Vicky was thriving on the placement, and I was just about muddling through, Ola's doubts about nursing had resurfaced.

One morning on the ward Ola confessed to me she was struggling with her English – which wasn't fluent – and that she continually felt tired. She was an animated girl but very unfit and her natural vim seemed to dissolve towards the end of a shift. Ola was further worried about her emotional attachment to the children. On her second day, a young girl with a diseased colon had a seizure in front of her. Ola had watched in horror, frozen, until the girl was stable again.

'I'm not sure I can cope seeing a child I'm caring for die,' Ola told me. 'I thought I could, but I'm not sure now.'

It's something we all had to ask ourselves, and I admired Ola's honesty. She was such a gentle soul and the young children really responded to her. But Ola was regularly battling her own emotions, and her fatigue – I had twice seen her in tears during shifts. I advised her to speak to Jenny.

For the last few days of our placement Ola didn't show up. Vicky and I later heard she had quit the course. We felt bad that we hadn't done enough to support her, but Vicky, ever pragmatic, said that if Ola couldn't survive a month on a ward then nursing probably wasn't for her. She had a point.

On the penultimate day of our placement it would be Julius's birthday. So far he had refused anyone visiting him except his medical team and his parents. This was understandable but Jenny finally persuaded him to see some classmates.

At first his friends, who stood at his bedside two at a time, were very awkward around him. But one of them, Obi, a chirpy basketball player with a crew cut, was completely uninhibited. He joked that Julius didn't have to go to school, could watch basketball on TV all day and was surrounded by hot nurses – except for me: 'that short, stubbly one'.

'You're living like a king, bro,' Obi said, looking around the room. 'Even got Beyoncé jiving about just for you.' For the first time in weeks, Julius smiled. It was shaky and short lived, but it was definitely a smile.

After Obi's visit Jenny took him aside. She asked him to get together a group of friends to visit on Julius's birthday. She also asked if Julius had a girlfriend. Obi said he didn't but there was a girl who was 'mad for him'. Jenny asked Obi to bring her along to the party.

I was starting to see Jenny's secret. In her eyes, everyone was a star. She told Obi that, with his honesty and wit, he could really help Julius out of a dark place. She told Julius's father he was a 'tower of strength' and his mother that she had 'the loveliest eyes'. She was like this with the staff, too.

Jenny's generous nature never felt fake. It helped create a good working atmosphere when she was in charge of a shift, making all of us keen to support our dynamic boss. So it surprised me that Jenny had not worked harder on cheering up Julius over the weeks. I asked her about this one day after handover.

'Think about it, Jimmy,' Jenny said, waving her hands at me. 'Julius isn't going to respond to an old bag like me. I told you he needed some space. I've given him that. I've watched him. Now he's ready. Just wait.'

It was fair to say Julius's birthday party could have been a disaster. His mother had made a cake for the guests, of which Julius couldn't eat a crumb, due to his tube-fed diet. The nurses all signed a card and sang him Happy Birthday. He was civil but didn't really perk up until Obi arrived with several members of Julius's old basketball team, and Hannah, a girl with long dreadlocks and a shy grin, who had a crush on him.

Julius stayed propped up on his bed. As a treat he was allowed four of his friends in the room at a time. I sat in the background, keeping an eye on things but letting them have fun. Soul music pumped out from a radio. While the others ate cake and joked around, Hannah sat on the edge of Julius's bed. With a gloved hand she tentatively stretched out, held Julius's arm and squeezed. They smiled at one another.

That afternoon something in Julius changed. All the anger and self pity of the past weeks seemed to pour out of him like creatures through a torn fence. His eyes welled at times but he just about kept control. Perhaps seeing his friends around him and feeling Hannah's touch, he realised he was going to be OK. Jenny, I thought, you're a bloody genius.

Over the next few days Julius was a different person. He was still in pain and knew he was unlikely to fully regain his fitness but he was tuned back into life. He asked about his treatment, how he could stay fit, when he could leave the hospital. He joked around with the nurses and his parents and Hannah, who continued to visit every day after school.

Despite the fact he might never play basketball again, the happy-go-lucky Julius in his bedside photo was back.

On my final day Snappy returned. The holiday had done little to brighten my mentor's spirits – she looked as mirthless as ever. Thankfully it was Jenny, not she, who was going to write up my final assessment on the ward. But Snappy wasn't done with me yet. She told me to accompany her to a quarterly discussion forum, where hot issues of the day were debated by the various members of the health team.

The first topic to be 'thrashed out' – Snappy's words – was whether it was a good idea for nurses to be able to prescribe drugs without supervision from a doctor.

Right from the start Snappy was blazing into one of the hospitals senior consultants, Dr Noble.

'Why on earth shouldn't we be able to prescribe drugs,' said Snappy, pointing her pen at Dr Noble. 'I've been a nurse for nearly twenty years. If I choose to up my skills – and my salary – by taking on more responsibility, why shouldn't I?'

Dr Noble (known as Dr No) cleared his throat politely. I'd seen him on the ward several times. He was a chivalrous, old-school doctor with ruddy cheeks and the sort of short, spiky beard once sported by musketeers.

'Cathy, I fully respect your argument . . . '

'I'm not sure you do . . . '

'Please give Dr Noble a chance,' said Rita, an occupational therapist (OT) who was chairing the discussion. OTs always made good mediators. Besides, you can't really argue with someone wearing an orange cardigan.

Dr No cleared his throat again. 'I just feel, Cathy, that doctors spend years studying human illness in great depth. It's our thing. Nurses are brilliant in many areas where doctors sometimes struggle – dressing wounds, injecting, empathetic care.'

'But we have good knowledge of drugs, too,' said Snappy.

'I don't deny it, Cathy, but you only study for three years or so. I have studied for over a decade, much of it specifically on medication. Of course a nurse could prescribe an aspirin for a headache, no problem, but what about the really complex stuff? A combination of mental and physical illnesses for example.'

'We could take extra courses . . . '

'But they are usually only a year long or less.' Dr No was primping his beard, something he always did when on edge. 'And if one nurse is able to prescribe, it opens the floodgates, which means it will put pressure on all senior nurses to be able to.'

'You're making it sound like us nurses are all dumbos.' Snappy raised her arms in the air as if worshipping some tribal idol. 'All hail the great Dr Noble, only he has the brains to cope.'

'Not at all,' said Dr No, calmly. 'I simply think that nurse prescribing is a way for the government to cut corners, cut costs. I think it will stretch nurses too far. I honestly do.'

I prayed Snappy wasn't going to ask my opinion because I agreed with a lot of what Dr No was saying. I had a lot of respect for him. He had a brain the size of Bolivia, but unlike some doctors was never superior, and spoke to his patients with a winning mix of compassion and clarity. He looked old enough to have worked alongside Florence Nightingale, and had served the NHS all his working life. He was a good man, who spoke good sense.

'I bet you are anti all us nurses having to get degrees too, hey,' said Cathy. She was clearly bristling for a fight. 'You think we're getting above our station?'

'My dear Cathy, I have no problem with nurses getting degrees,' said Dr No. 'No problem at all. That's your business, not mine – but nurse prescribing greatly affects me.'

At this stage a woman called Mrs Morgan, one of the hospital managers, walked in. She was dressed to the nines in an executive suit, with shoulder pads jutting out like a Super Bowl quarterback. She slumped down in the seat next to Dr No, the whole room soon overwhelmed by her musky perfume. Dr No, in his corduroy jacket and ancient shoes, looked to be from a different planet altogether.

'Sorry I'm late, I've been at my son's school,' said Mrs Morgan, plonking down her briefcase. 'Do you want me to update you on how the hospital renovation is going?'

'We're on nursing degrees at the moment,' said Dr No, giving her an encouraging smile. 'The fact nursing might soon become an all-degree profession. I think it's a good thing. Midwives already need degrees, so do physiotherapists and occupational therapists. Why not nurses . . . '

'I disagree,' Mrs Morgan interrupted. She was clearly no fence sitter. 'I think scrapping diplomas for nurses is a bad idea. Certain nurses won't be able to afford the degree. It will mean nurses will only come from the middle classes. They won't want to get their hands dirty.'

'I resent that comment, Mrs Morgan,' said Snappy. 'I have a degree, and I still empty bedpans. Just because someone has a nursing degree doesn't make them too posh to wash.'

'No,' said Mrs Morgan. 'But it will make you more keen to become a manager or a senior nurse . . . '

'Well, why shouldn't I?' snapped Snappy. 'Nurses are allowed to seek promotion just like anyone else, aren't they? You may get a great salary, Mrs Morgan. Well, I don't.' Snappy was angry now, well, angrier than normal, her cheeks flushed a ripe shade of burgundy. 'I'm not bitter or jealous or anything. I like being a nurse. I accept nurses need to empty bedpans and wash patients. Of course they do, it's a caring profession. But why shouldn't all nurses get a chance to move up the career ladder? It's a job with a lot of responsibility and it's time that was understood.'

'But what about those who can't afford to do a degree?' repeated Mrs Morgan. 'Only diploma students get a full bursary.'

'I think money should go to those who can't afford it,'

Snappy said. 'There are huge dropout rates on nursing courses. A degree-only system might stop this. I think anyone who has what it takes to be a nurse, whatever their background, should get the funding . . . '

'I think you are being idealistic,' said Mrs Morgan.

'Well, I don't,' replied Snappy. 'Nurses who don't want a degree can become health care assistants.' Snappy stuck up her chin defiantly. 'If health care assistants were trained and paid better it would be a more appealing job than it is now. They are truly the unsung heroes.'

'How would you pay for all this, Cathy? The NHS has more than 400,000 nurses. Even a small wage rise would be hugely expensive.'

'By paying us doctors less!' joked Dr No, trying to hold out an olive branch to Snappy. 'Oh, dear me, what a tricky topic. Degree or not degree, that is the question. And it's a very hard one.' Dr No was gamely trying to lighten the atmosphere but Snappy was having none of it.

'I don't think we should pay nurses any less – or doctors either,' she stressed. 'We should slash the NHS financial consultants both in wages and numbers.' She made a chopping gesture with her arm, nearly hitting Mrs Morgan in the eye. 'And we need to cut down litigation – the NHS loses more than one billion a year on bloody law suits. And hospital car parks should be free . . . '

'And pigs might fly,' said Mrs Morgan, under her breath.

'And so might you, Mrs Morgan,' said Snappy. 'With shoulder pads like that.'

Mrs Morgan looked stunned. She was relatively new to our team and I sensed nobody had spoken to her like that before, let alone a nurse. There was a thin line between being critical and being plain rude. Snappy had just crossed – make that leapfrogged – that line. The silence was so heavy you could drink it.

'I think Rita's got more chance of flying in that splendid cardigan of hers,' Dr No said softly. He winked at Rita and began to laugh. We all tentatively joined in. Good old Dr No, always the diplomat.

'Let's stop it there with the degree debate★, ladies and gents,' said Rita, slapping the top of her legs as a gesture of finality. 'Mrs Morgan, why don't you give us your update on the hospital renovations . . . '

After the meeting Snappy seemed pretty pleased with herself. To be honest, she had impressed me – by both her knowledge and her passion – but I told her I thought she'd been a bit hard on Dr Noble.

'Oh, Dr No knows I'm an awkward sod,' Snappy said, as we walked back through the hospital garden. 'He never takes it personally. He's old school. I agree on most things with him, but can happily hurl a bit of abuse, too. He doesn't mind.'

Snappy sighed and explained that Dr No had been around since the early days of the NHS, when doctors were all called 'Sir' and patients respected everything they said. She said it was not like that now – the media criticised doctors, patients swore at them – but unlike many of his colleagues, Dr No had dealt with these changes with good grace.

'And what about Mrs Morgan?' I asked.

'Oh, she's all right for a manager,' said Snappy, shrugging. 'She might talk like she's got a melon up her arse, but she works hard and cares about the hospital. Just needs to lose a bit of ego.' Snappy grinned. 'I just wanted to ruffle her feathers today, that's all. She needed that. We nurses don't speak up enough.'

★Nursing is to become a degree-only profession by 2013, and the diploma will be scrapped. In my group roughly a third were doing the degree, the rest the diploma. We all spent equal amounts of time on the wards, but the degree coursework is a little more academic.

To be fair to Snappy this was true. Over time I noticed nurses often didn't fight their corner with doctors or managers. They preferred to stay quiet or toe the line, doffing to the doctors' medical knowledge, when often it was they who knew the patient far better. Of course, there were the likes of Snappy or Mr Temple, nurses who always forcefully put across their point of view, but they tended to be the exceptions.

Back at the ward Snappy needed to head off to another appointment. She glanced through my nursing portfolio and signed off my final time sheet.

'Sorry I haven't been a very good mentor to you,' she said. 'Not really my thing. Jenny tells me you didn't do too badly.' She shook my hand with the formality of a duchess. 'Good luck, young man.'

Snappy hadn't been the easiest mentor, but it was clear she cared both for the ward and the nursing profession as a whole. Her no-nonsense brassiness and Jenny's cheery dynamism had made my first month as a student nurse one to remember.

Later that evening, once Vicky and I had said our farewells to everyone on the ward, we met up with Jana in a local bar. Jana had enjoyed her placement, too, but had been jolted by a particularly tough final week, when a baby on her ward had died. She had visited the morgue with the parents and had seen the coffin, 'not much bigger than a shoe box'.

We were all strangely subdued. Vicky and Jana looked pensively into their drinks. It seemed we'd all grown up a lot over the last few weeks. Then Vicky said she wanted to go to McDonalds and I point blank refused and Jana called me an old git and a Madness song started playing on the jukebox – and we all had another round of drinks, and then another and, just for a while, everything was all right with the world.

Chapter 6

MIDLIFE MAYHEM

I had three days off before my next placement – vital time for ironing my uniforms and catching up with Jess, family and coursework. It was becoming clear that being a student nurse was a juggling act. You jitterbug between three different worlds – the wards, academic study and your personal life.

In many ways I had it soft. Other than teaching the odd private English class to foreign students – for which I could set the hours – I was free to focus on the nursing. But several of my fellow students were not only training to be nurses but working like Trojans in shops, cafés, pubs and offices. One adult nurse, a towering Geordie called Kevin, had even enlisted as a special constable. He later plumped for the police full-time, joking that he was: 'Good Cop, Bad Nurse.'

Others had family responsibilities. In our group Coco helped care for a father with Alzheimer's, Vicky cared for her autistic sister, Sheena had a new grandchild, and Evaristo, a mental health nurse, quite literally had a football team of a family, with seven children and four grandchildren.

My family responsibilities were light. My parents were both healthy. My daughter Poppin, who had been such a big part of my life, was overseas. I spoke to her regularly and made financial contributions, but my role was hardly hands-on.

It was Jess who kept me on my toes. She was something else. She encouraged me to exercise, to practise CPR and the obs, to hit essay deadlines, to always do my best. Despite her busy work schedule I was touched that she still found time to occasionally iron my uniform or make me packed lunches. At times I wondered if she was borderline bionic.

Jess was a human dynamo, no question, but this could prove exhausting at times. We seemed to be having far too many conversations that went something like this:

Jess (while watching a mountaineering documentary about some hearty, snow-crusted hulk, ice-picking his way over the Alps): 'You know, Jimmy, I've always wanted to climb Mont Blanc.'

Jimmy: 'Me, too.'

Jess (excited): 'Really?'

Jimmy: 'No, not really, too tame. K2 is more my kind of mountain.'

Jess: 'You're joking.'

Jimmy: 'Yes.'

Jess: 'You're such a slouch, Jimmy. Will you ever climb any mountains with me?'

Jimmy: 'The Brecon Beacons – as long as I can take a hip flask and a full team of sherpas.'

Jess: 'It's a deal. But no sherpas. It will be good training for Mont Blanc.'

Jimmy: 'You're joking?'

Jess: 'No, I'm not. And all the exercise will reduce your nursing-induced tension.'

Jimmy: 'Nursing-induced tension? What's that? Sounds serious.'

Jess: 'Fatal. But I will cure you. We start training tomorrow.'

Jimmy: 'Great. Just in time for me to buy some Kendal mint cake and a bag of steroids.'

(Jess bounds up the stairs two at a time singing 'Climb Every Mountain'. Fade out.)

To help unleash nursing-induced tension – as Jess so eloquently put it – she enlisted me in a group called British Military Fitness (BMF): perhaps the ultimate in midlife crisisdom.

BMF is run by ex or serving army members and is a cross between a gym class and a boot camp. It is always held in the open air, whatever the weather. This suited me fine. I can't stand the soulless nature of gyms – the tortuous machines, the muted TV screens and all those muscle-bound posers. Give me the sun, the rain, the snow – or at least that's what I thought.

Jess attended the first BMF class with me. Before setting off into the park our group of forty or so were handed out different coloured shirts by the instructor, a khaki-clad beefcake called Joe The shirt colours were green for the super-fit, red for the semi-fit and blue for the newbies, smokers and dossers. Jess, naturally, joined the greens and I, rashly, joined the reds. The shirts were numbered, too. My shirt was Number Seven. David Beckham, eat your heart out.

It all started off very gently. Lots of jogging slowly in a circle while whirling our arms around. This is going to be a breeze, I decided. Even John Prescott could do this. After ten minutes, though, things got serious. The greens, reds and blues split up. The reds all had to charge across the park at full speed and then dive on to the ground whenever Joe shouted: 'Grenade!' Oh joy! By now it was near dark and the recent rain had turned the ground to sludge, caking us in mud.

After this our filthy group was made to stand underneath the branch of an oak tree. 'Jump up and grab hold of it,' barked Joe. 'Go on, jump up like a monkey!' I jumped up but, being a short arse, couldn't reach the branch. 'What are you like, Number

Seven?' The next thing I knew Joe had grabbed me by the arm-pits and was lifting me up to the tree. The ultimate humiliation. I managed about two and a half pull-ups and then collapsed. 'I said act like a monkey, Number Seven, not a sloth!'

It got worse. After several more sprints and dozens of sit-ups and push-ups, we were ordered to run up a steep hill. This in itself was a Herculean challenge, but, to up the ante, we had to piggyback someone at the same time. I tried to pair myself off with a svelte-hipped girl – about a third of the reds were women – but ended up with a stocky bruiser called Matt. Before I could suggest Matt carried me – he looked a lot younger and stronger – he had jumped on my back. 'Tally ho,' he shouted. Plonker.

Matt weighed a ton. I staggered halfway up the hill. Then came that glorious sound: 'Grenade!' I discarded Matt and collapsed in the damp grass, panting like a spaniel. Now it was Matt's turn to carry me. I mounted, hands on his sodden shoulders. My weight seemed to make no impact on him at all. He set off, as fleet footed as Hawkeye in *The Last of the Mohicans*, zigzagging up the hill. But nearer the top his pace faltered and he asked me to jump off. He paused, gasping, gesturing for me to carry on without him. Up ahead Joe shouted: 'Grenade!' and we all hit the deck again. I swear, if any mental health nurses had been watching we'd have all been sectioned immediately.

After everyone got up I realised Matt was still lying face down on the ground. 'Matt! Matt!' No response. Joe and I rushed over and checked his respirations. He was ashen faced, his breathing strained but regular, his pulse jittery but distinct. Thank God, no need for the kiss of life or a rendition of 'Nellie the Elephant'. We gave Matt some water and made him lie on his back, elevating his head under my trainers and his legs on a nearby tree.

Soon he regained his colour and we joined the rest of the group back at the car park. Matt explained he was anaemic and had very low blood pressure. At times this caused him 'to swoon' if he hadn't eaten properly or if his blood sugar was low.

Or, let's face it, if he'd just run up a stonking great hill with me on his back.

Even though Matt's situation had been far from critical, and my intervention hardly life saving, it was the first time I had put my nursing skills to any sort of use outside of the hospital. It felt good.

Matt ate a chocolate bar while I did some stretches with the rest of the reds. Matt told me he was a greenkeeper at a local golf course and had suffered from depression for years. He'd tried endless pills and therapies, but found BMF to be the best remedy of all.

'I do it three or four times a week,' he told me, as I stretched my hamstrings on a gate post. 'I've met a great bunch of people. It livens me up, you see – unlike bloody golf. I couldn't last a week without BMF now. The instructors are the best.'

Personally, I could last whole lifetimes without BMF. I felt like hell – damp, cramped and physically shot. But I also realised Matt was right – there was a great sense of camaraderie within the group. And yes, I had to admit it was wonderful to feel my blood fizz again. I'd never have pushed myself this hard in a gym.

After the stretching Matt headed for the pub while I joined Jess who had just finished her session. 'Wasn't that great!' she said. She looked as though she could do it all again.

'Let's meet Jenny and Fred at The White Lion,' she suggested, wiping some mud from my face. 'It's quiz night.'

'I can't, sweetheart,' I reminded her. 'I'm on an early shift tomorrow.'

'Just for a little while,' she replied, blowing me a kiss. 'All this military fitness will keep you going. And don't forget, we're hill racing on Sunday.'

I wish I hadn't gone to the quiz night at The White Lion. The following day was my worst nursing shift to date, and I should have been at my most alert.

It was my second day of the new placement, working alongside

Hadia, who was my student companion this time. We were on a children's ward specialising in orthopaedics and neurology. Many of the children were either recovering from operations or waiting to go under the knife.

The ward was run by Sister Josephine, a brusque, efficient Irish woman, with humour as salty as dry-roasted peanuts. When she saw me her response was: 'Ah, here he is, the token male student.' And when she saw Hadia: 'Ah, here she is, the token student in a headdress.' Luckily, Hadia took the comment in her stride. I found Sister Josephine refreshingly un-PC and, although not as warm as Jenny, still capable of running a tight and happy ship.

The dozen children on the ward ranged from babies to sixteen-year-olds. There were three children who had been in car crashes, including a Down's syndrome toddler with a bad head injury. One teenager was hoping for corrective surgery on her bowed legs and there were several children with breakages, including a Bengali boy in traction with a fractured thigh.

But on that particular shift, all our attention was on Sally.

Sally was a sixteen-year-old schoolgirl whose punky hair and attitude belied a crushing insecurity. She had recently jumped off a bridge in a suicide attempt. Her right fibia and tibia – the two major bones of the lower leg – had been shattered, her skin severely degloved and her spine damaged. She was known to drink heavily and had been diagnosed with both bulimia and depression. Her parents had recently gone through an acrimonious split, a possible trigger for her jump. Sally continually told the nurses she wanted to die.

Even though teenage suicides are rare,* Sister Josephine was very concerned about Sally. She explained to Hadia and me that

*Young suicides are always tragic but they are decreasing. Around 24,000 young people aged between 10–19 attempt suicide each year, the majority of them female. Only about 1 in 50 die. The biggest current rise in suicide rates – up 15 per cent over the last few years – is in the 35–64 age group.

more women attempt suicide than men, although many more men actually succeed, and in the UK at least three times more men die by suicide than women.

But Sister Josephine felt that Sally's chosen means of self harm – a bridge jump – was a more masculine approach and, therefore, potentially more worrying. Whereas men tended to use a weapon, hang themselves or jump from heights, women tended to overdose, often ineffectively. Sally's bridge jump might well have killed her. The fact she was a heavy drinker was another vulnerable trait for the suicidal. For this reason she was on permanent observation.

Sally was tricky to deal with, and Hadia and I, as callow students, were advised to stay clear of her. The cubicle curtain around Sally's bed was usually drawn shut, but we often heard her fire insults at the nurses tending her. 'Leave me alone!' 'What's your problem!' 'Just let me die!'

Early that evening Sally's father visited the ward. Mr Smith was a boorish-looking man with elaborate tattoos all over his forearms. He smelt of alcohol and stale sweat. He was bristling over the fact that the operation on Sally's leg, due to take place that afternoon, had been delayed.

'So sorry, Mr Smith,' said Hadia, the first member of staff to speak to him. 'The surgeon had to deal with an emergency. Sally will be operated on tomorrow.'

'You people,' said Mr Smith, pointing his podgy finger in Hadia's face. 'Letting my little girl lie there all afternoon, worried out of her skull.' He continued to swear horribly about Hadia and surgeons and the NHS, unconcerned about young children being in earshot.

Sister Josephine had already gone home, and a gamine, soft-spoken nurse with auburn hair called Alexa was now in charge.

'Please, Mr Smith,' said Alexa, putting up her palms to placate him. 'We are terribly sorry. We will do our best to get Sally operated on as soon as possible.'

'Not good enough,' shouted Mr Smith.

'Please, dad,' Sally called from her bed. She was in tears. 'Pleee-ase, don't do this.'

'Shut up, Sal, you don't understand. They've let us down. Messed us up big time.'

'We are only trying to help,' said Hadia, showing great courage. 'Please don't disturb the other children. You are behaving very badly.'

There was a pregnant pause. Mr Smith looked like thunder, a vein on his forehead pulsing.

'Who's this fat, fucking bitch?' shouted Mr Smith, pointing at Hadia, but addressing Alexa. 'What right has she got to tell me to do anything. After this I'll track her down. Track her down and . . .'

'That's enough,' I said, as Hadia, stung by Mr Smith's cruel tirade dashed to the nurses' station. 'I'm calling security.'

'Fuck you, shorty,' spat out Mr Smith, jabbing his finger at me. Alexa moved between us.

'No, Jimmy, don't call security,' ordered Alexa, seemingly more angry with me than Mr Smith. 'I've got this under control. You are a student. Unable to deal with this. Wait in the station.'

I'm not a violent man at all and would be a dead loss in a fight. But never in my life had I wanted to headbutt somebody so much – Mr Smith, that is, not Alexa, although I would have liked to have given her a good shake, if only for her to see sense and call security.

I knew my raging anger at Mr Smith was utterly inappropriate. As nurses we are supposed to have a quality called Unconditional Positive Regard. It's a phrase coined by the American humanist Carl Rogers, back in the fifties, meaning we should give everyone the benefit of the doubt, be non-judgemental. I'm sure Mr Smith had a thousand reasons for behaving in such an unspeakable manner, but I couldn't help but judge him. Anyone who swears violently in front of young children and threatens a teenage nurse was just plain nasty. I wanted him out of the ward, preferably dragged by his collar. If not, I would happily fell him with a bedpan. But, I had to remind myself, I was still a student. A middle-aged student, maybe, but I still had to defer to experience.

In disbelief at Alexa's judgement I joined Hadia at the station and made my shaken colleague a cup of tea. I then watched the unfolding events through a glass panel.

Anyone could see Alexa was way out of her depth. She kept apologising to Mr Smith, trying to console him. In many situations this would have been a good approach, the sort of thing a textbook tells you. But Mr Smith was beyond this, he had thrown all the books out of the window. This was not a time for soft skills. Mr Smith was boiling over, artery popping, inconsolable. It didn't matter what Alexa said, what any of us said, he wanted retribution and nothing would get in his way.

The stand-off between Mr Smith and Alexa went on interminably. Alexa, almost a foot smaller than him, cooing away like some dove of peace, and Mr Smith, a raging Yahoo, chewing up the furniture. Both were so puffed up, they had forgotten the fear and chaos they were stirring up around them.

To make myself useful I left the nursing station and tried to comfort Sally, who was now in a state of hysteria. The young Bengali boy in traction in the bed next door was being consoled by his father. A tranquil, cool-headed man, he stroked his terrified son's hair and read him a fairy tale while Mr Smith and Alexa played out their war.

Mr Smith was now becoming more physical, kicking at the floor and hitting his fist into his palm. He perhaps sensed Alexa's proud façade was fragile and wanted to break her. I knew two security guards were on permanent standby just outside. I had seen them earlier when I'd escorted a child to surgery. The guards could have come in at any time and defused the situation. Alexa remained convinced her communication skills would win the day, unaware that Mr Smith had stopped listening ages ago.

Events soon spiralled further out of control. Mr Smith's verbal abuse was becoming increasingly loud and toxic. He kicked a child's plastic chair, which flew across the ward in a blur of orange. Several of the children were now crying. The situation was out of control.

'Stop it, dad!' yelled Sally from her bed. She was a freckly girl but had gone so puce with anger and embarrassment that all her freckles had vanished. 'Stop it!'

But Mr Smith continued to harangue Alexa. Finally, one of the other nurses, Martha, a self-assured Polish woman, increasingly frustrated with Alexa's leadership, called for security. Two large men in black uniforms walked in. Mr Smith, confronted with these hulks, lost all his bombast as fast as a punctured balloon.

To keep face Mr Smith groused a bit more about the NHS being hopeless, but, deprived of nurses to bully, he soon surrendered to the physically superior guards. Like most bullies, deep-down Mr Smith proved to be craven. As he was escorted out he called to his daughter: 'Sal, I'll be back, you hear, girl, I'll be back.'

Poor Sally wept hard and loud, like some wounded animal. God only knows what home life she'd had to endure with a father like that.

An hour later Hadia, Martha and I walked out of the hospital after having attended a debrief about the Mr Smith incident.

'I can't believe how rude he was,' Hadia said, as we stood at the bus stop. 'I've never been spoken to like that before. He made me cry, the horrible man.'

'Yeah, it's no fun being called a fucking bitch,' said Martha, unfurling her umbrella. 'If it helps, when I worked at A & E I was called much worse.'

'Oh, *that* didn't bother me,' replied Hadia. 'But he called me a fat bitch, too. *Fat*! That's what made me cry!'

At this we all began to laugh uproariously. I really took my hat off to Hadia. Only nineteen, fresh out of the family home, living in a grotty nursing hall, grappling with a new city and now threatened by a foul-mouthed thug: it impressed me she was still laughing. At the beginning I thought Hadia would be one of the first to drop out. I'd got her all wrong: she was a trouper.

Mr Smith visited again the next morning but was not allowed into the building. He sat musing on a bench in the hospital garden. After a grovelling apology note and some negotiations with Sister Josephine – if only she had been on duty that night this would never have happened – Mr Smith was granted permission to accompany Sally to surgery that afternoon. He remained strictly banned from the ward though.

At handover Sister Josephine told Hadia she could accompany Mr Smith to the operation. Seeing Hadia's jaw drop, Sister Josephine burst into laughter. 'Only joking, my love,' she said, winking. 'You've already paid your dues.' Hadia looked bemused. She was having trouble grappling with our boss's waggish sense of humour.

'So, Jimmy, being the token bloke,' said Sister Josephine, flicking through the ward diary, 'you can go. You connected well with Sally last night and if Mr Smith gets upset he's less likely to insult you.'

'Less likely to insult me!' I protested. 'He told me to f-off, shorty.'

'Oh, I'm sure you've heard worse than that,' said Sister Josephine, brightly. 'You've got that look about you. A face to launch a thousand quips.'

'How kind of you to point it out, Sister Josephine!'

'Besides, it's good experience, Jimmy,' she added. 'Accompanying patients to theatre is often a student's job. It would be a real help.'

And so at midday, accompanied by Harry, the hospital porter, an elderly but tough-as-boots ex-soldier, we wheeled Sally off to her operation. Mr Smith was still waiting outside in the hospital garden. He looked bashful, a baseball cap pulled low over his eyes. He'd shaved and put on an ironed, long-sleeved shirt. He scrubbed up pretty well.

'You Mr Smith, my friend?' said Harry, ever friendly but with the natural authority of an ex-military man. Mr Smith nodded.

'Follow on then, sir.'

'Thank you.' Mr Smith shook Harry's hand. 'Thank you so much.' Mr Smith moved straight over to Sally, who lay on a gantry swathed in blankets, her head propped by pillows.

'I'm so sorry, love,' said Mr Smith, grasping Sally's hand. He held it as if it was the most precious thing on earth. 'I was drunk yesterday. Made a fool of myself. I'll be fine today. I love you, Sal. Love you so much.'

Sally, after an unsuccessful attempt at looking gruff, broke into a huge smile. 'It's OK, dad. I love you, too.'

We rattled Sally down endless corridors. The gantry was unwieldy to push, like a supermarket trolley with the wheels kinked in the wrong directions. Surgery took place in the hospital basement and the whole area was lit by spectral, jaundiced lighting. We finally reached the anaesthetist's room. It was clear Harry knew them all. In fact Harry seemed to know everyone in the hospital whether anaesthetists, receptionists, nurses or consultants. Wherever he went there were greetings: 'Hi, Harry!', 'Afternoon, Harry', 'Good on you, Harry', and: 'Still not dead yet, Harry?'

In turn Harry greeted all the anaesthetists. 'Hello, George, how's the new baby, keeping you awake at night?' 'All right, Sandy, I heard you did a skydive, you mad bugger.' 'You've put on some weight, Carmen, suits you, girl.' Thank God he hadn't said that to Hadia.

The anaesthetists were a close-knit group full of in-jokes and well-oiled banter. I imagined it was important to stay upbeat living in this twilight world, cooped in its permanent gloaming. Carmen – the one who Harry had complimented on her weight – came out to talk to Sally and Mr Smith. She was a middle-aged woman of Colombian descent with dark hair, an easy smile and a voice full of music. Her scrubs were spotless, emblazoned with the name of the hospital, and she radiated a calm confidence.

Sally was becoming nervous. Carmen looked directly at her with grey, dancing eyes and told her what to expect. She explained how Sally would 'go under', then have a complex operation that would fuse her shattered bones. Carmen used soft, clear, comforting language and Sally soon relaxed. The NHS had so many superb people like Carmen and Harry and Sister Josephine. One could not help but feel very proud sometimes.

Mr Smith gripped Sally's hand like a lifeline. He was quiet today, a different man to the fire-spitting savage of last night. The anaesthetist's procedure was so slick, that in no time Sally was looking drowsy, then sleepy, then gone under.

Mr Smith watched her calmy, kissed her tenderly on the fore-head and walked out of the room. I followed him into the foyer and held back as he stuck some coins in one of those heavy-duty coffee machines. Coffee was a good idea for Mr Smith: Sally's operation was due to last several hours. The machine wheezed and clunked and spewed out dark froth.

Mr Smith took the cup and sat himself in one of the blue plas-tic chairs you often see in hospitals, linked together like modern church pews. I sat next to him. When I looked over, I noticed tears rolling down his face.

'Don't worry, Mr Smith,' I said. 'They'll do everything they can for Sally. She's in the best of hands.'

'It's just . . . ' Mr Smith put down his coffee and wiped at his eyes with the back of his hand. 'It's just that moment. You know. When Sally went under. It's like she's gone from you, and you can't do nothing.' He dabbed at his eyes again. 'Like, you know, her soul's leaving her body.'

Mr Smith was in a state of high emotion, his body shaking as if ravaged by a tropical disease. I briefly rested a hand on his shoulder.

'I'm sorry,' he said, grimacing with tears. 'This is embarrassing. Crying like a fucking baby.'

'It's very natural,' I assured him. It was, too. I'd accompanied several parents to see their loved ones undergo operations. Minutes before they might be joking around, everything's going to be fine, cocksure. But when the anaesthetic kicks in, when the eyes flicker, the face drops to one side, and their beloved child is rolled off through the perspex double doors and into a strange, dimly lit world ruled by strangers in blue pyjamas, tears will often fall. In that moment even the biggest Jack the Lad, the sturdiest earth mother, will drop their mask and pray.

After recovering himself, Mr Smith wanted to talk. Talk and talk. As a student nurse I found that this often happened, near strangers spilling their life story. Being a middle-aged male nurse people didn't know what to make of me. Over time on the wards I got mistaken for a doctor, a pastor and a cleaner, and, while out in the community, without my uniform, I was regularly seen as a builder. At times this hard-to-pinpoint quality made me approachable.

Mr Smith talked about how much Sally meant to him – 'my whole world, mate, everything, *everything*!' He talked of how he'd loved his wife, how she'd suffered from depression for years. Self-harmed a bit. He didn't mind, though. She was the most beautiful woman he'd ever seen and he still loved her, still stuck by her. 'I didn't care about the tears, the tantrums,' said Mr Smith ruefully. 'What a sucker.'

It turned out Mr Smith's wife had later left him, sloped off with one of his best mates. She'd gone to live up north and lost all contact, started another family. Left Sally and him in the lurch. Mr Smith said the anger and shock had almost killed him. He couldn't cope, started drinking and lost his job as a labourer. Sally couldn't cope either. She started skipping school, drinking and giving Mr Smith lip.

'I slapped Sally once and hated myself,' admitted Mr Smith. 'Never hit her though, never, ever. She's my life.'

Around this time Sally had started self-harming. She tried to make contact with her mother, but she never replied to Sally's letters. On the phone her mother was civil at first, but then more and more aloof. Sally stopped trying, got herself a punk haircut and kept skipping school without her father knowing. Mr Smith found work in a scrapyard in the day, and a supermarket at night. He stopped drinking but he was hardly ever home, wanting to earn money to help Sally's future. He'd organised for Sally to see a counsellor at school and thought she was doing OK. Next thing he knew she'd jumped off a bridge.

'When I was told about her suicide bid I was sick.' Mr Smith was spent now, his tears dried, the zip in his voice gone. 'Physically sick. To think I hadn't been there for her. Hadn't noticed how miserable she was. How messed up she'd been by her mother, by me. She seemed the strongest of all of us but, well, she's just a little girl . . . ' His voice cracked and his eyes welled again. There was a long pause while he got it together.

'Last night I was bang out of order,' Mr Smith whispered, fiddling with a crucifix around his neck. 'I'd not drunk for weeks. I took the afternoon off work to be with Sally for the op, then got the phone call about the cancellation. I just flipped.' He clicked his fingers. 'Couldn't hack it no more. Drank about a bottle of fucking whisky. I was wild, out of control.'

'You're not joking,' I said.

He slapped his head and rummaged around in a plastic bag at his feet. He pulled out a box of Heroes chocolates. 'That poor girl I shouted at, Christ I'm ashamed. Can you give her these for me.' I was about to tell him he should do it himself, but then remembered he'd been banned from the ward.

'Yeah, sure, I'll give them to her.'

'Thank you, mate,' he said. 'And thanks for listening. I bet that's the worse fucking case of midlife crisis you've ever heard.' It certainly made my worries about BMF look pretty tame.

'Was I rude to you, too?' asked Mr Smith.

'Very,' I said. 'I cried all night. You called me shorty.'

At this he let out an explosive laugh, and I laughed, too. I don't know how much of Mr Smith's story was true but it certainly sounded pretty convincing. Having loathed the sight of him last night I had to concede I now rather liked, even admired him. I'd made a snap judgement that he was a brutal thug. I'd forgotten one of the most basic rules of nursing – that people are not always as they seem.

I left Mr Smith praying for his beloved Sally. He was looking down at a dog-eared photo of her he kept in his wallet. He'd asked me to leave him and was now alone in the waiting room, his face tight with anxiety. Watching him sitting there, I imagined others like him in hospitals all over the world. Thousands of people touching photos, twisting wedding rings and kissing amulets: all of them fumbling in the darkness for a talisman of love.

Chapter 7

YINING AND YANGING

I checked on Sally first thing the next morning. Her operation had gone well, and she seemed much calmer than usual. She told me Mr Smith was due to visit later. 'He's a great dad really,' she told me, as I headed over to handover.

To my surprise, there were two other male nurses sitting in the nurses' station. On a children's ward to have three male nurses all working together is highly unusual.

'Ahoy there,' said the younger and larger of the two. 'Another bloke, another one of us.' He had shaggy blond hair and skin that looked as if it rarely saw daylight. 'I'm Stan and this', he pointed at a cherry-faced, bespectacled man sipping on a coffee, 'is Joe.'

Joe looked up and smiled. 'I should add,' he said, blowing on his cup, 'that both Stan and I shatter the stereotypes of male children's nurses. We are both straight.'

'How can you say you're straight, Joe,' interrupted Martha in her strong Polish accent. 'You like Duran Duran.'

Joe laughed and began to sing a deeply flawed version of 'Rio': 'Her name is Rio and she dances in the sand . . .' before being heckled to be quiet by a couple of nurses who had been on the night shift.

'Martha has a theory that you can judge a man's sexuality by his music tastes,' explained Joe, rifling a hand through his short, greying hair. 'She likes heavy metal, so God only knows what that says about her. She's probably got more testosterone than all of us put together.'

It's true that many people still perceive male nurses to be gay. As soon as I announced I was going to be a nurse, certain friends – admittedly, the more uptightly macho ones – asked me if this meant I was gay. As if by becoming a nurse, this immediately changed my sexuality overnight. In reality, of course, some children's nurses are gay, and some are not. I'm sure there's some statistics somewhere but I couldn't really care less if someone's gay or straight – or if someone thinks I'm gay or straight: unless I'm on a date with them.

'So, Joe,' said Martha, while reading a patient's file, 'tell us your favourite three bands. I already know Stan's, and they are pretty butch. Stuff like Johnny Cash and the Clash.'

'Oh, that's easy,' said Joe, putting on a high camp voice. 'They would have to be . . . Barbra Streisand, Celine Dion and Kylie.'

'Whey hey, he's all man, this one,' shrieked Martha. The rest of the nurses whooped with laughter, except Hadia who looked completely confused by the whole conversation. 'You big tease, Joe. I know you like the Rolling Stones.'

'OK, for real this time,' said Joe, scrunching up his eyes. 'It would have to be . . . the Stones, the Kaiser Chiefs and Robbie Williams.'

'You hang in the balance, Joe,' decided Martha, peering over her glasses like a TV judge. 'Bit of yining and yanging going on. Stones – yanging, Robbie – yining.'

When it was my turn I admitted to Bruce Springsteen, the Beatles and the Dixie Chicks. According to Martha, I had a bit of yining and yanging going on, too.

'But the Dixie Chicks are bad-ass rockers,' I said.

'No, Jimmy, Led Zepellin are bad-ass rockers,' replied

Martha, doing a passable impersonation of Jimmy Page air guitaring. 'And maybe Guns N' Roses, Jimmy Hendrix. But not,' she tut-tutted, 'the Dixie Chicks.'

Martha explained she based her theories about sexuality on the Kinsey reports, conducted back in the 1950s in America. Dr Kinsey suggested that only 10 per cent of people are totally heterosexual and 10 per cent totally homosexual, the rest lying somewhere in between.

Hadia, who until then had been quiet, made an eloquent but rather stark announcement. It centred on her religious beliefs: the fact that the Koran predicts that there will be nine signs that the world will end, one of them being more homosexuality.

'Some of the signs are obvious,' added Hadia, straightening her headdress. 'Things like global warming. But others are more subtle, like men becoming more feminine.'

'You mean like male nurses,' said Stan, looking a bit angry.

Hadia sensibly paused to think about this. 'Well, nursing historically has been a woman's role. But being a nurse doesn't necessarily make a man more feminine.' Good answer, Hadia, I thought, in that it didn't say anything. She'd make a great politician.

'That's nothing to do with it,' said Martha. 'It's due to a decline in male fertility. Very different to male virility. No disrespect to your religion, Hadia, but the gayest of men can shoot out babies like there's no tomorrow while the biggest heterosexual hunk can fire on blanks.'

Hadia shook her head at this point, but Martha continued: 'Roughly one in a dozen men are now sterile and the number is rising.'

'How do you know that, smart arse?' interrupted Joe.

'Genes fascinate me, big boy,' replied Martha, squeezing Joe's leg. 'It's down to sperm creation in the male Y chromosome becoming faulty. It means increasing numbers of males can't reproduce. Men might even become extinct one day.'

'Bring it on,' said Barbara, a world-weary agency nurse sitting in the corner.

But according to Martha, there was hope men wouldn't die out. She'd read an article about the mole vole, a creature that lives in the mountains in Central Asia. She claimed the mole vole had, somewhere down the line, lost its Y chromosome but was still able to reproduce by transferring its 'maleness' genes to a separate chromosome.

'Martha,' said Joe, winking, 'you'd better transfer some of your Motorhead genes to make up for my Robbie ones.'

Sister Josephine walked in at this stage and handover began. 'Three male nurses on one shift!' she noted, innocent of the conversation we had been having. 'Watch out, ladies, men are taking over the nursing world.'

It was fair to say that men did seem to dominate aspects of nursing, especially the management. Indeed, the Chief Executive at the Royal College of Nursing, and perhaps the most prominent voice of nursing in the UK, is a man called Peter Carter.

Male nurses also tend to win better pay deals, being twice as likely to secure high-ranking jobs, despite women often being better qualified. One reason for these discrepancies is that female nurses, many of them also mothers, are much more likely to go part-time at some point in their nursing careers (around 50 per cent), compared to only 5 per cent of male nurses.

On our ward, though, Sister Josephine was definitely Queen Bee and deservedly so. But, for my first and only time as a children's nurse, I was to have a male mentor – Stan, whom I had already met at handover. Hadia, who also hadn't been allocated a mentor yet, was given Martha.

During my opening days with Stan it was clear he never got rattled by anything. He was a gentle giant who had trained as a welder, but after attending a nursing open day at a local college with a friend, he had decided to switch careers. He'd gone on to qualify as a nurse, while his mate, who had initially been interested in nursing, became an estate agent.

'My mate's sold his soul,' said Stan, grinning. 'But he doesn't mind. He's making shitloads of money.'

Stan was particularly good at teaching clinical skills, no doubt helped by years of tinkering with broken car parts. As I am the king of the cack-handed, I was often grateful for this.

One clinical skill that is essential to master as a student nurse is the taking out of cannulas. These are minute plastic tubes that are inserted into a vein so that the medication or liquid can go straight into the bloodstream. Putting in cannulas is usually a job for doctors. First a needle is injected into the vein, and once the blood starts running, the tube is stuck in.

A student nurse never usually inserts cannulas but spends a lot of time removing them. Although intimidating at first it's not a difficult job. After the first weeks on the ward, under Stan's guidance, I had become pretty slick with cannulas – but then I had to deal with Aldo.

Aldo was an Anglo-Italian toddler with Down's syndrome, who had suffered a head injury as a result of a car crash. Aldo was a good-natured lad and the staff all loved him. But when he was unhappy – boy did you know about it.

I had got to know Aldo and his family well over the last days. They were a large, amiable bunch, who would crowd around Aldo's bed and, true to their Italian roots, all talk at once, gesticulating like impassioned stock traders.

Aldo was on a cocktail of drugs, some received via a cannula in his arm. He was also fed by a naso-gastric tube as, like many Down's syndrome children, he had problems with digestion due to an underdeveloped oesophagus. Stan had taught me how to clear the tube of air bubbles and carefully monitor its flow. By feeding Aldo, giving him medication, and helping him dress in the mornings, I had built up a good bond with him.

But then disaster – I needed to take out Aldo's cannula. I

prepared a tray with the usual kit: gloves, sterile wipes, a plaster, some cotton wool. At first Aldo was fine, and lit up with a big smile when he saw me. But as soon as he realised I was after his cannula, he began to wail. He wouldn't let me near him. Normally, I could easily calm Aldo when he was upset, but this time he was inconsolable.

I decided to leave him for a while, and ask for Stan's advice. Stan listened quietly and then said: 'Jimmy, sometimes you have to be cruel to be kind. This is a clear case of JFDI.'

'JFDI?' I asked.

'Just fucking do it,' said Stan. 'Aldo always has a problem with cannulas. Best thing is to act fast, and then it's over with. Don't prolong his anxiety.'

Stan also advised me to call on the services of Rebecca, the play specialist. Before starting with the NHS I had never heard of play specialists. Their title says it all – they are at hand to play with the children. It sounds the most flaky role imaginable, like filling the ward with the cast of *Teletubbies*.

But play specialists are much more than just a perky presence, although I have to admit that Rebecca, with her purple jumper and Alice band, did look a bit like an escapee from a 1980s *Blue Peter* episode. Yet for all her persistent jollity Rebecca was a pro. When not on the ward she would regularly visit A & E to ease children overcome with fear and pain. She was a valued member of the team.

Rebecca suggested we took the portable TV over to Aldo's bed and play *Shrek*, his favourite film. Once she had distracted Aldo sufficiently, I honed in on his cannula. JFDI, Stan had said, and that's what I did. Aldo moaned briefly while I pulled out the tiny tube, wiped away the blood spot and put on a plaster. It was all over in seconds.

Afterwards I thanked Rebecca for her help. She pointed out that play specialists are the only people on the ward the children have no agenda with. Surgeons, doctors, nurses, physios and psychologists all have to deal with things children don't like much – pills, syringes, washing and health warnings. But play specialists simply play, something all children like to do.

'My job is hard to justify on paper,' admitted Rebecca. 'And some of my friends laugh about it. But I know I'm doing good work and that's what counts.'

When I asked Rebecca if she'd ever met a male play specialist she laughed and said: 'You must be bloody joking!'

Something extraordinary happened late one afternoon. A Russian woman, sporting chestnut hair and fancy clothes, came into the ward with a tiny baby, no more than a month old. None of the senior staff nurses were around and there was a fair amount of confusion as the woman spoke no English.

For a while the young mother sat looking in wonder at the walls of the ward. This, to be fair, is what most people did when they first came in. The walls, I should explain, were painted purple with a lurid selection of jungle beasts on a backdrop of wilderness. Lions, tigers, monkeys, snakes, coconuts and mangos all vied for her attention. Many children's wards go in for this type of *trompe l'oeil*, but I had never seen walls quite this mind-boggling. The Russian lady, who looked to be no more than twenty years old, seemed so distracted that she fell into a trance, while rocking her son to her chest.

Stan, calm as ever, gauged the situation. He finally gestured for the mother to put the baby on one of the spare beds. He then asked me to phone around and track down a Russian interpreter.

I should explain the variety of cultures on the ward was wildly diverse and several of the children did not speak English as their mother tongue. In the nursing station a long list of more than thirty interpreters was on display – Bengali, Albanian, Urdu, Swahili – and, thank God, Russian.

I got through to an interpreter called Ivan who said he could be with us in an hour. While all this was going on, things were busy on the ward. Sally, who had made good progress since her operation, was undergoing physio, Aldo was having a tantrum and another child with a leg brace was being admitted. We were also very short of staff.

After securing the interpreter I prepared Aldo's food. A few minutes later Stan tapped me on the shoulder.

'Have you seen the Russian woman, Jimmy?'

'No,' I replied. 'What's up?'

'I think she's done a runner,' he said, cool as ever. 'And left us with the baby.'

Stan asked me to search the ward thoroughly, including bathrooms and storerooms, then to check the neighbouring wards, the hospital garden and the canteen. I dashed around like fury but nobody had seen her. Within the hospital, her trail had gone quickly cold.

'Oh, bollocks,' said Stan, when I got back. 'This is looking bad. Check the surrounding streets and bus stops, Jimmy. You might just find her.'

I tore off into town. It was wet and cold, the evening sky full of indistinct stars. I sprinted from one bus stop to the next, poking my head in any cafes and shops en route. The young mother would be easy to spot as she had been wearing a hat made out of something large, grey and hairy.

After twenty minutes running around, asking a few startled bystanders if they'd seen the runaway Russian, I gave up. I hoped she'd decided to return to the ward. As I was walking back towards the hospital, lost in thought, I heard a deep, vaguely familiar voice shout my name.

'Is that Jimmy? Jimmy Frazier?'

A man in a dark suit jogged up to me. It was John, someone I had been at school with years ago.

'What the hell are you doing here?' he asked. 'And what are you wearing?' I realised that in my haste I hadn't taken off my uniform or my student nurse badge.

'I'm looking for a missing Russian girl,' I said, sounding like a character from *Spooks*.

'A missing Russian girl?' asked John. 'Are you a pimp or something?' Clearly I didn't sound like a character from *Spooks*.

We gave each other a brief update on our careers. John proudly informed me he now worked in advertising. He couldn't believe I was a nurse, and asked if I had turned into 'some sort of nancy boy'. Here we go again, I thought.

'So you must snort cocaine and talk bullshit all day,' I replied. 'Isn't that what advertising folk do?'

We exchanged a bit of gossip about our contemporaries and agreed that we should meet for a drink sometime. John was a likeable bloke but I sensed our worlds were now far apart. Seeing him did get me thinking, though, as I walked back to the hospital. Here I was, emptying bedpans and dashing around trying to find Anna Karenina, while he had just sealed a lucrative deal for a new ad campaign.

I suppose I might have been doing something similar, donning a suit, sealing deals and drinking espressos. And some days – usually the ones when I had been shouted at, or had witnessed something awful – I did question what I was up to. But, for all that, working on wards was never boring. And, on the good days, the rewards blew everything else out of the water.

Back at the ward the Russian mother was still AWOL. Sitting with the baby were Stan and Ivan, the interpreter – who in my haste I had forgotten to cancel. He was a jolly, barrel-chested man with a black beard, who said he would stay on call for whenever the mother returned. Fortunately, he wouldn't have to wait long.

The Russian mother, whose name we now discovered was Tatiana, returned early the next morning, looking far less elegant. In fact she looked like a little girl lost, gaunt and scared, with her big blue eyes bloodshot. Incredibly her baby son didn't seem to have missed her at all, and had slept well during the night.

Tatiana explained to Ivan that her Russian lover, a wealthy businessman, had fled the country due to corruption charges. She was completely alone, and hadn't a clue what to do. She knew hardly anyone in the UK.

She had entered the hospital on a whim, and then, realising the baby would be safe on the ward, scarpered. She had spent the night in a cheap hotel, and now, despite looking well dressed, was almost broke. She'd wanted to leave her baby son at the hospital as she didn't feel capable of looking after him, but guilt had driven her back.

The baby should never have been on our ward in the first place and was soon moved to another, while Tatiana's mental state and social circumstances were looked into. With uncharacteristic tetchiness Stan announced: 'We've got enough on our plate without looking after some oligarch's moll.' I was glad to note Stan, the king of composure, could become frazzled at times, too.

That same morning Aldo was due to have surgery on his oesophagus to enable him to eat without the use of a naso-gastric tube. Aldo was constantly in and out of theatre, either to clear the clot on his brain following his car crash, or to sort out his digestive system.

The emotional toll on his family was tough. Compared to Tatiana's *laissez-faire* attitude to her baby, Aldo's mother, Christina, a delicate-looking woman with long dark hair, was at her son's side whenever possible. She was as protective as a lioness and told me she had been since Aldo was born, having heard that more than 10 per cent of Down's syndrome children die within the first year of their lives.

But Christina had always believed Aldo would survive. Even though he had problems with mental retardation, weak muscles and poor digestion, his heart, often a problem for children with Down's syndrome, was relatively strong. Medical advances had also worked wonders. Indeed, the average Down's syndrome life expectancy is now over fifty years.

'I'm just sad he'll never have his own children,' said Christina, before we headed off to surgery. 'Very few Down's syndrome men can reproduce, although the women can.'

'It's not all bad though, is it, my love?' added Christina, kissing Aldo on his nose. 'Down's syndrome means he's got much less chance of developing certain cancers and his arteries are less likely to clog up, too.' She patted her stomach and smiled. 'Unlike Mum's arteries, hey, Aldo – too much parmesan!'

Medicine confounded me sometimes. What sort of strange evolutionary justice meant Down's syndrome could prevent certain cancers and yet cause Aldo so many other problems? But Christina liked to look on the bright side.

'God gives with one hand and takes away with the other,' she said, as we steered Aldo towards the surgeons. 'I'd like to think Aldo understands that. He seems such a happy child despite everything.'

I'd asked Stan if I could watch some of Aldo's surgery, which he'd agreed to, as had Christina. Having transported Aldo to the anaesthetists, I made my way to the surgeon's changing area – a huge, dank-smelling locker room in the basement. Here I donned a set of blue scrubs and a pair of plastic sandals – the standard surgeon's garb.

I flip-flopped my way down a Stygian corridor and eventually reached theatre. In a side room I was asked to put on a lead jacket. I took one hanging from a rail and draped it over my head. I felt like a medieval archer sporting a tabard, but to protect me from X-rays rather than arrows. The jacket felt very heavy – the weight of a damp and baggy trench coat.

It was a different world here in Surgery Land. The clothes were different, as was the language, and even the music: something classical as opposed to the easy listening of the wards. Aldo, stretched out on a black table, was unrecognisable. A white sheet covered him, except for his upper chest, the focus of the operation. Not seeing his face gave the event a necessary, impersonal quality.

Aldo's surgeon, Mr Todd, a craggy, silver-haired man, made his first incision. I was immediately in awe of the responsibility surgeons have to deal with every day. Of course, I knew this already, but seeing surgery live really hits it home – what the likes of Mr Todd do is nothing short of dazzling. One wrong call, botched cut, failed stitch, and a child might die. No wonder surgeons have a reputation for arrogance, I thought. They really are playing God. Strangely, when I had NHS operations as a child, I always remembered my surgeons as rather avuncular, a far cry from the ego-pumped preeners on the TV shows.

Mr Todd seemed assured, if a bit brusque with his assistant, a young female trainee. His hands were now dark with Aldo's blood as he delved into the young boy's insides. He constantly asked for fresh surgical tools, which the nurses would bring over to him.

Theatre nursing is a very specific skill and, although not squeamish, I didn't like the idea of it much. The only real contact a theatre nurse seemed to have with patients was when they were knocked out on the operating table. Sure, an encyclopaedic knowledge of surgical tools and keeping a cool head were no doubt vital – plus not pissing off the surgeon. But I had come into the profession to communicate with patients, and this intense, quiet, twilight world did not appeal at all.

I watched the operation for half an hour. From what Mr Todd was saying, it sounded as if there were several complications and Aldo would need further surgery.

Back in the ward I bumped into Christina who asked me how Aldo's operation was going. I played my dumb student nurse card and said it wasn't clear yet. Someone more skilled could spell out the bad news later. Christina was with Aldo's younger sister, Pippa, a little girl dressed up as an angel and sporting a tinsel halo. Christina wanted to take Pippa to the canteen, so, as it was the end of my shift, I agreed to escort them.

I took them via a short cut, past the entrance to A & E, which proved a big mistake. Usually this would be fine, but today some paramedics were offloading a stretcher with a seriously injured young cyclist on it. The cyclist was deathly pale, his blond hair soaked with bright, congealed blood. The paramedics were shouting instructions, one of them holding an oxygen mask to the cyclist's face. I noticed Christina automatically crossed herself and said a silent prayer as she looked on.

'Silly bugger hadn't been wearing a helmet,' I overheard one of the ambulance drivers say to his colleague. 'Youngsters think they are immortal. Sodding tragedy.' Within the hospital setting it was well known that helmet-free cyclists were known as 'brain donors'.

I quickly ushered Christina and Pippa past the ambulance. But we weren't clear yet. Slumped against the A & E entrance was an elderly man, with a shock of white hair and a face caked with dirt and vomit. He was wildly drunk and smelt foul. A couple of nurses were trying to move him on and he was swearing horribly, calling them everything under the sun. When Christina came into his view he reached out towards her: 'Hello, gorgeous. Come here, I won't bite you.' Christina shrieked, grabbed Pippa, and dashed ahead.

'Just run off then, you bitch,' yelled the old man. 'You're a horrible bitch, just like the rest of them.'

'I'm so sorry,' I said to Christina, as we finally chicaned our way to the canteen. 'I was trying to take you by a shortcut.'

'Don't worry,' she said. 'Stuff happens.'

I could see Christina's face was tense, but poor Pippa looked shell-shocked. They didn't deserve this at all. God, what a mess.

And soon Christina was likely to be told Aldo's operation hadn't been a success and he'd have to go through the whole thing again. I wondered how long she could maintain such grace.

'You can have a nice drink now,' Christina said to Pippa, trying to comfort her. 'Maybe have a cake? An ice cream?' Pippa was becoming tired and weepy. Christina enveloped her in a big hug. 'Let's be strong for Aldo, honey pie.' The little girl was still dressed in her angel outfit, her tinsel halo poking out above her mother's arms.

This was no place for angels today, I thought. And, for all Christina's silent prayers, there didn't seem much of God around, either. Feeling guilty, I suddenly desperately wanted to get away.

That evening, I pedalled home furiously. There were shifts like this sometimes, when enough was enough. The speed of the bike felt good. Here was power at the click of a gear, speed at the turn of a pedal. It was all so simple. And if anything went wrong my bike could always be fixed. Tinkered with, greased, welded, panel-beaten back in shape, sorted out. How unlike the frail and complex human engine.

On our final day at the ward Hadia and I presented Sister Josephine with a box of chocolates. 'Ah, the token box of chocolates,' she said, somewhat predictably.

Hadia had also made Stan some flapjacks. An uncomfortable frisson had existed between the two of them from the start when Hadia had hinted that nursing was an effeminate profession. Stan, the ex-welder, hadn't liked this or Hadia's religious doom-mongering and, although never rude, he often gave her a wide berth.

I was impressed that Hadia had picked up on Stan's irritation and now wanted to make amends. Hadia was clearly from a strict Muslim background, and often had her nose in some sort of Islamic text. She also prayed regularly. Being away from home for the first time, she was being challenged on so many levels.

She'd been threatened by Mr Smith, insulted by Mr Temple and must have found the ribald banter in the nurses' station tricky. But she was making every effort to adapt.

At the end of the shift Hadia and I said our goodbyes to all the nurses and the children. Aldo had made us both cards, which Christina handed to us. Mine had a dinosaur on the cover – I think I still have it somewhere.

That evening Stan, Joe and I had a few pints together. It was a good opportunity for me to ask them if they had ever considered another branch of nursing other than children's. Didn't they get fed up being men in a woman's world?

'I've always found women more interesting than men,' mused Stan, swigging on a lager. 'As a welder all the blokes talked about was cars, sport and girls. Three top subjects, no question, but the conversation got a bit repetitive.'

'Women talk so much crap though,' insisted Joe. 'I love them to pieces, but sometimes I really need to get away from them.'

'Oh, me too,' agreed Stan. 'But in the workplace I have no problem being around women. They tend to be more competitive with themselves than with me.'

'I never try to be one of the girls, Jimmy,' said Joe, munching on a crisp. 'Being a male nurse it's important to be yourself. Look at things from a male perspective.' He laughed. 'And yes, do stuff like barbecue steaks, drink beer and talk football now and then.'

'While listening to Robbie Williams,' said Stan. 'You hard bastard.'

'The yin and yang, bro.' Joe drained his pint. 'But the main reason I do this job is because I love kids. And because I'm damn good at it. That's all that really matters. Sod what anybody else thinks.'

I'd enjoyed my children's nursing so far, and hadn't felt too alienated being in such a female dominated profession. I knew that at the end of the first year we could switch to either adult or mental health nursing – both had more male recruits – but I hadn't ever seriously considered it yet.

'Did you know Florence Nightingale disapproved of male nurses, Jimmy?' said Stan. 'Yup, the Lady with the Lamp decided their "hard and horny" hands shouldn't tend the wounded, no matter how kind their hearts.'

'Oh, well,' said Joe. 'You can't win them all. She might have thought differently today. Besides, my hands aren't hard and horny. I even moisturise.'

'Steady on, Rambo,' said Joe, laughing. He raised his glass. 'One thing's for sure. We male nurses need to stick together. All for one and one for all, fellas.' We clanged glasses and promised to stay in touch.

Chapter 8

BEDPAN BLUES

It was about this time that I split up with Jess. Beautiful, lion-hearted, high-octane Jess.

I remember the night clearly. We had arranged to meet at military fitness and I'd arrived late. It was already dark by the time I got there. I locked my bike, put on a red shirt and charged after the rest of the group. I was struggling to catch up. I cranked up my speed to a full-blown sprint but still the other runners were way ahead. In the paltry moonlight it was all I could do to keep them in eyeshot. What was wrong with me? This was something I would normally find easy.

'Number fifty-six!' I heard Jess shout from behind me. 'What are you doing? That's the local athletics club. We're over here!'

Panting and humiliated, I jogged over to my usual group. I had mistaken the athletics club, who also ran in red shirts, for BMF. Jess thought this hilarious and ribbed me mercilessly. After our session we both walked hand in hand through the park to a neighbouring pub. The rich, woody smell of bonfire smoke was in the breeze.

Our drink started off joky and affectionate but the atmosphere between us soon became strained. It didn't help that the pub was so crowded we had to shout to make ourselves heard above the happy-hour din. In short, Jess accused me of not spending enough time with her friends (true) and not understanding her work (true). I accused her of not understanding my work either (true, but at least she tried).

Following one final heated exchange – this centred on my lack of enthusiasm for an Iron Man contest somewhere in Yorkshire (swimming, cycling and running absurd distances) – she slammed down her wine glass and walked out, her final insult, 'You are a man of tin, Jimmy', still ringing in my ears. On the plus side it was better than being a man of straw. But, whether a man of tin, iron, straw or flesh and blood, it was clear my relationship with Jess was now wrecked, smashed against the rocks, scuttled. After a subsequent row on the phone we agreed to call it quits.

In truth, this moment had been looming for some time. I could blame it all on Jess's thirst for daredevilry, but actually my increased focus on nursing played a far bigger part, as did my inability to commit to anything more than a few weeks ahead.

We had been together for almost a year. Despite having had some brilliant times together, we were now veering in wildly different directions. Jess was fast scaling the greasy pole of promotion at work, while most of her leisure time was spent training for her ever more pulse-quickening physical challenges. She was a great girlfriend, but in terms of our future plans, we were not meant to be.

Like most break-ups, it was far more painful than I imagined it would be – even with the added relief of not having to climb Mont Blanc. Jess and I agreed not to speak to each other for several months. I missed her sorely and, as a palliative to my bruised heart, plunged myself into the nursing.

My renewed focus on the course was good timing as I had an important OSCE exam looming.

I had no idea what OSCE stood for – still don't, come to think of it – but I knew it was vital for me to pass it if I was to continue my nurse training. Mr Temple described it as 'the big one'.

The OSCE is not a written exam but one that assesses your practical skills in strictly timed conditions. A group of clipboard-wielding examiners – including Mr Temple and Super Nurse – would watch us do such things as take blood pressures, check urine samples and carry out CPR. The thought of accurately taking Mr Temple's pulse in exam conditions was truly terrifying. The man was practically cold blooded, for heaven's sake. Like one of those sub-tropical lizards, he could probably stop his heart at will.

Many of our group were anxious. Even Vicky and Coco, usually the coolest of customers in pressurised conditions, were in a funk. Jana was 'bricking it', Hadia and Shima were praying to Allah more than normal and Sheena was convinced she had already failed the course for scoring low marks in her coursework to date.

It was fair to say Sheena was struggling. As a grandmother in her fifties, with a brace of fresh grandchildren to help care for, she had a lot on her plate.

Sheena, by her own admission, had little idea how to construct essays or use computers. She was, however, a battler. Despite struggling with her written work she was a star turn on the wards – compassionate, hardworking and capable. And yet, without ticking all the academic boxes, this would count for nothing.

I wondered about the logic of this. Of course nurses need to master some classroom theory before hitting the wards and, yes, the discipline required to complete the written work was important. But I felt Sheena had other qualities that would make her a top-class children's nurse, and far eclipsed her lack of academic nous.

Further striking terror into Sheena was the fact that, as future nurses, we all needed to pass the strangely named European

Computer Driving Licence (ECDL), which consisted of seven 45-minute computer exams. Seven! This had been sprung on us at very short notice and the shock of it was too much for Sheena.

The day before the OSCE she decided to quit. 'I've loved every minute,' said Sheena, embracing us one by one. She was clad, as always, in one of her vibrantly coloured African dresses. 'But the coursework is too much. It's unfair on my family. I've got no choice but to leave.'

This was a blow for all the survivors. Sheena was the oldest in the group, a solid and inspiring presence. With her gone, our initial posse of students had now been halved. I wondered if by the end of the OSCE there'd be any of us left at all.

The OSCE was the first exam we needed to attend in a uniform. We had been told by Mr Temple to 'scrub ourselves up' to make our practical tasks seem as authentic as possible.

I met up with the rest of the group, all immaculately turned out in neat blue tops, in the exam room. The next few minutes would determine whether or not we made the grade as nurses, and the anxiety was evident. In fact, we resembled victims of an imminent firing squad.

Super Nurse appeared and told us we would each have our own patient, who would be lying in a hospital bed. Within ten minutes we needed to accurately record their blood pressure, pulse, respirations and temperature. Thank God the patients were strangers, I thought, which at least meant they wouldn't be Mr Temple.

I was first up, along with Shima and Hadia. Shima was so nervous she was shaking all over and Hadia was unusually quiet. Super Nurse, with her comforting, megawatt smile, ushered us each to our individual beds. My patient was an athletic-looking black teenager with Afro hair and a lopsided grin. I introduced myself and discovered her name was Lea.

The examiner watching us from the end of the bed was a stern lady with half-moons specs, wielding a clipboard. She looked like Cruella de Vil.

Before starting my observations on Lea, I had to wash my hands. This was also a test. Hospital-acquired infections – many of them due to poor hand washing – cost the NHS over a billion pounds a year and contributed to thousands of patient deaths. So hand-washing tests, however absurd and Monty Pythonesque they sound, were important.

Cruella nodded to show I had washed my hands sufficiently. Thank God; to have failed my degree due to a grubby mitt would have been too humiliating for words.

I returned to Lea. First up, I felt for the radial pulse on her wrist. My hand was shaking and I couldn't trace any pulse at all. Oh, God. I began to sweat. Cool it, Jimmy, you can do this. Cruella looked on, unimpressed. I felt again. Nothing. Jesus, don't panic, man. You've done this in hospital a thousand times. Come on, this is the one. Don't screw up. Then yes, yes, yes! There it was, Lea's pulse, pumping good and slow. Phew! This relaxed me. I even threw Cruella a cheeky smile, before continuing with Lea's temperature, respirations and blood pressure. I wrote down my readings as Cruella scribbled on her clipboard.

'That's it, young man,' said Cruella, after a quick debrief. She peered at me over her half-moon spectacles. 'Go on, off you go.'

I got up, thanked Lea and washed my hands once more. As I made to leave Mr Temple came up and gently tapped me on the back. 'Well done, Jimmy. Good work. I had my doubts about you at first, but you're going to be fine.' He smiled, a genuine smile, as opposed to one of his usual pinched, joyless ones. He even told me to have a good weekend. He seemed a different person altogether – breezy, larky and almost cool. Stunned and rather pleased with myself, I walked out into the hospital forecourt. It was windy, with rain ripping into the earth like gunfire.

I dashed for cover under a sheltered archway, where I bumped into Hadia and Shima.

Shima was in floods of tears. She'd apparently struggled to find her patient's pulse because her hands had been shaking so much. She'd panicked and completely messed up the rest of the exam. Hadia was reassuring her friend that she would have a second chance, and would be less nervous next time.

A few minutes later Vicky, Jana and Coco came out of the exam room. They all seemed pretty upbeat but played this down when they saw Shima's distress. Hadia signalled for us all to move on and leave her and her distraught friend in peace. We ran through the rain back into the hospital cafe and sat by a radiator to warm up, our clothes steaming.

'Poor Shima,' said Vicky. 'That was a scary exam.'

'God, yeah, I was so nervous,' said Jana, sipping on her tea. 'When I was holding the thermometer, my hand was shaking like crazy. Mr Temple was my examiner. He took hold of my wrist and told me it was all OK. Told me to relax.' She flung her head back and laughed. 'I couldn't believe it. Mr Temple calming me! Anyway, he held me until I stopped shaking. And then I was fine!'

I related Mr Temple's generous words to me, too. Coco said she had heard Mr Temple was always hard on new nursing recruits up until OSCE time. Rumour had it he only acted like a devil early in the course in order to weed out those students not dedicated enough.

'You know what,' said Jana, smiling, 'I'm beginning to think Mr Temple's a bit of a sweetie.'

'You should give up this internet dating lark,' teased Vicky. 'Take a chance on Mr T.'

'Maybe I will! Me and Mr . . . ' Jana paused, rubbing her forehead in thought. 'I really must find out his first name. He's like Batman or Inspector Morse – we never get to know it. Adds to the mystery though.'

'Whey hey, this is getting serious!' shouted Coco. 'Jana and Mr T. I think I can hear wedding bells.'

'Mr Temple would certainly have interesting wedding vows,' I said, pretending to put a ring on Jana's finger. 'She will be mine. All mine!'

'Ah, shut up the lot of you,' said Jana. 'You're all just jealous.'

'I certainly am,' I admitted.

I told them my relationship with Jess was over. My lack of stamina and her devotion to yomping across deserts and jumping out of aeroplanes had finally taken its toll.

'You can always surf the net for love, Jimmy,' suggested Jana. 'I could help you with your profile.' She paused to think, rubbing her chin. 'How about this – male nurse, all own teeth, likes running around parks piggy-backing strangers, rants endlessly about modern society, happy to meet anywhere – except Starbucks, looking for a Dixie Chick to twang his heartstrings.'

'And his purse strings,' said Vicky.

'And his ding-a-ling,' said Coco.

I scrunched up my napkin and threw it at her. 'I've been hanging around you girls far too long,' I said. 'Thank God we're back on placement next week.'

The following Monday I began work on an adult ward. Despite specialising in children's nursing we were encouraged to spend time experiencing other disciplines. The ward turned out to be one of my toughest experiences as a student nurse, but I'm very glad I did it.

The ward was huge, with thirty beds, and run by two separate teams of nurses. I was in Team B, where most of the patients had vascular (relating to blood vessels) problems.

As a student nurse you often get a gut reaction about a ward during the initial handover. On this ward I didn't get so much as a gut reaction as a full-blown gastro grenade. Even before the handover the omens were not good. All the nurses sat in silence, kicking their heels and looking glum. Sure, it was 7 a.m. and everyone was a little bleary, but for nurses to remain mute at any time of day was rare.

To compound the feeling of unease most of the staff seemed to be agency, with little idea about the ward. I had no named mentor, but was taken under the wing of another student nurse who was in her third year. Her name was Sam, a tall, straight-talking Cockney in her mid-forties. She told me she had worked on the ward before and had requested to come back.

'Biggest mistake of my life, sweetheart,' whispered Sam after handover, tying up her long ginger hair. 'This ward used to be great, with a lovely sister. Now it's a disaster. No one has a clue what's going on. Just not enough nurses. It's amazing what a difference a year makes.'

Sam was helpful but too busy to give me much advice. She asked me to help care for three patients, who all shared the same bay. There was snow-haired Ron, a war veteran in his mid-eighties, missing his right leg at the knee. His left leg was also swollen and threaded with angry blue veins.

In the far bed was Jack, a portly ex-merchant seaman recently out of heart surgery. There had been complications and Jack had spent several weeks bed-bound. He now had severe ulcers on both his legs, which needed regular dressings. In the middle bed was Malcolm, a gaunt and stubbly student, who was temporarily in the ward, recovering from an appendectomy.

That morning it was my job to do the observations on Ron, Jack and Malcolm, feed them and help with their personal hygiene. I'd had very little instruction, so decided to just get on with it.

The ex-soldier Ron was my first patient. On top of all his other ailments he had suffered a stomach upset in the night and needed a commode at repeated intervals. There was no available hoist but Ron's delicate frame made him easy to manoeuvre. He always maintained a merry, stiff-upper-lip attitude, despite his wretched condition. The merchant seaman Jack was also easy-going, and called all the nurses 'captain', whether male or female. His leg ulcers must have been agony, but he was forever cracking jokes, even during wound dressings.

Sam had warned me that both Ron and Jack, in their jeopardised states, were vulnerable to blood clots. Clots were thought to cause a staggering 1 in 10 fatalities in UK hospitals – roughly 500 people a week – more than road accidents, HIV, breast cancer and MRSA combined. Yet, despite both Jack and Ron receiving anti-coagulant drugs, they seemed to have little idea what they were for. From the chaotic state of the ward, I sensed there was very little time for thorough, empathetic care here, let alone the handing out of advice.

And yet, compared to 21-year-old Malcolm, who was in mild discomfort from his appendectomy, Ron and Jack were a picnic. Malcolm spent his time yabbering on the phone to his friends, swearing loudly. He would think nothing of pressing his red emergency buzzer on the flimsiest pretext. One time I was midway through helping Ron on to a commode and had to leave in order to dash over to Malcolm, who had been frantically pressing his buzzer.

'Nurse,' whimpered Malcolm, who only minutes before had been in rude health, 'I've got hiccups.'

I could have throttled him. I'd stopped assisting a fragile octogenarian to rush to the aid of this whinger. I took a deep breath, smiled, fetched Malcolm a glass of water, and rushed back to Ron. My reserves of unconditional positive regard soon started to erode with Malcolm. Throughout the day his continued swearing and moaning really began to grate.

Ron's daughter and grandchild, a young girl of about ten, came to visit him that afternoon. The old soldier's face lit up with delight. At the same time, a grungy-looking friend of Malcolm turned up sporting a studded dog collar. I have no problem at all with how people want to dress but I do have a problem with their attitude, and this ghastly pair continued to swear and boast of their sexual conquests, unconcerned they were in easy earshot of Ron's young grandchild. Malcolm's lack of respect towards the elderly servicemen was disgraceful, and I increasingly wanted to confront him.

While I was dressing one of Jack's wounds later in the afternoon, Malcolm's red buzzer once again sounded off. I apologised to Jack and rushed over.

'Nurse,' Malcolm groaned, rubbing his stubbly chin. 'Make me a cup of tea, will you.'

That was it. I was exhausted and for the first and only time as a student nurse I lost my temper with a patient. It wasn't professional, it wasn't clever, but, my God, it felt good. I told Malcolm that his friend, who was leaning back on a chair reading *Heat* magazine, could have got his tea. In fact, he could have got it himself. Malcolm was due to be discharged the following day, and had been mobile for some time, but, when in the company of health professionals, he always acted as if he was on his deathbed.

Once I had begun my tirade I found it hard to stop. I told Malcolm he had shown a complete lack of respect to Ron, Jack and their families.

'And as for the red buzzer,' I pointed at it for emphasis, 'that is for emergencies. For your information hiccups are not an emergency. Tea is not an emergency. You have taken me away from a very important job, to help you do one you could have easily waited for. Frankly, you are leaving tomorrow, and should start taking responsibility for yourself.'

I paused and took a few deep breaths, realising I had not only overstepped the line, but, as a student nurse, hurdled it. 'I'm sorry I've talked to you like this,' I said, more softly. 'And I am more than happy to help you when you need it, but right now, the gentleman in the next bed to you is my priority. So put that in your pipe and smoke it.' Actually, I didn't say that last bit, but

Malcolm still looked suitably aghast. And, despite some killer stares in my direction, he never swore, pressed the red button, or even hiccupped again, until his merciful discharge the following morning.

Working on the wards really had the capacity to surprise me sometimes. So far, despite seeing some emotionally charged situations, I had always felt in control. I thought, perhaps due to having my own young daughter, it would be working with very sick children that would upset me the most. But no, what finally tipped me was caring for Mr Prosser.

Mr Prosser was in an isolation unit and suffering from advanced gangrene in his left leg. The damage caused was now drastic – his skin blue-black from shin to toe – and his lower leg was likely to need amputation. His foot was so dark that from a distance it looked like coal, but on closer inspection it was more the texture of black pudding, damp and congealed. It also reeked. I had been asked to assist a junior doctor take off the antiseptic dressing, which only covered part of the gangrene, and inspect the wound.

Most of the junior doctors I had worked with to date I had found very caring with their patients. They also seemed confident – but not Dr Jerrams, who was only recently qualified.* He was one of those uptight people whose eyes could never settle and who spoke in an uppity 'haven't got all day' manner.

Dr Jerrams began by unwrapping and checking a fresh sterile dressing kit at the foot of Mr Prosser's bed. The kit was packed in a white box, a bit like a present. Having impatiently removed the various items – dressings, sterile wipes – Dr Jerrams snapped

---

*Every August, 50,000 junior doctors start work or begin new rotations in the UK. Hospital deaths rise by 6 per cent in the week that follows. Thankfully, I was unable to track down any similar statistics for newly qualified nurses.

on his plastic gloves. He then perused Mr Prosser's leg, squinting down at it, his nose almost touching the ruined skin where the existing dressing did not cover.

'I need a bedpan, please,' Mr Prosser whispered. He directed this request to me. I had got to know Mr Prosser well over the last few days.

'Not now, Mr Prosser,' said the doctor sharply. 'I need to crack on and get your leg inspected. Won't take long.'

'But I need it now,' Mr Prosser stressed, his face a picture of discomfort. 'Please, I honestly do.'

'Not now, please,' Dr Jerrams repeated. He was clearly not taking in a word his patient was saying. 'Now move over, Mr Prosser, so I can get to this leg. Help him, student, will you.' I listened in disbelief at the way this coltish upstart was speaking to Mr Prosser, bossing him around as if he was ten years old. I wasn't thrilled at being called 'student' either. I will be forever grateful that Sam came in at this stage.

'I think Mr Prosser needs a bedpan,' I told her immediately.

'It can wait!' fumed Dr Jerrams, a premature fogey if ever there was one, Sir Lancelot Pratt trapped in the body of a man in his mid-twenties. 'I'm in a hurry. Need to get this leg done.'

'Please help me,' implored Mr Prosser in an increasingly shaky voice.

'I'm getting a bedpan now, doctor,' said Sam firmly. 'Mr Prosser needs it. I can easily do his sterile dressing if you need to go.'

Dr Jerrams looked at her in disbelief. He was clearly not used to being upstaged by a student nurse, albeit a formidable middle-aged one with Michael Caine specs and ginger hair.

'If you have a problem with that,' said Sam, smiling icily, 'I'll tell the sister.'

Dr Jerrams knew when he was beaten. 'Very well,' he said, attempting to preserve some face. 'I'll let you get on with the dressing and I'll come and inspect the leg later.' Dr Jerrams snapped off his gloves, threw them into the waste bin and marched out.

Sam winked at me and rushed off to get the bedpan. I was really impressed by Sam's authority. She had worked as a health care assistant for years before training as a nurse, and it put her in good stead. She was one of the most competent nurses on the ward, despite still being a student.

When I looked down at Mr Prosser I noticed he was crying. He looked utterly miserable. 'I'm sorry, I'm so sorry,' he said, tears streaming down his cadaverous face, his grey stubble as bristly as pine needles. 'I couldn't wait for the bedpan. I've messed myself.' He turned away from me. 'I'm so sorry.'

'Don't worry, we'll clean you up in no time, Mr Prosser,' I told him.

'I want to die so much,' he said quietly. 'Right now. Join my Maureen. My lovely Maureen.'

I had spent quite a bit of time with Mr Prosser over the last few days and he had spoken of his wife non-stop. They had married when both were in their early twenties, and apart from Mr Prosser's stint in the army during the war (he had been wounded in North Africa), they had never spent a day apart since. They had no children, but had run a successful laundry business together for over forty years. Reading between the lines, Maureen had clearly been his whole life, and when she had died of cancer two months previously, Mr Prosser had given up the will to live. He had been found in his flat, bed-bound and near to death, his leg already beyond repair. Since then he had been stuck in this gloomy isolation room. Whenever I had cared for him, he spoke only of Maureen, and of wanting to die and join her.

When Sam came back, we both cleaned up Mr Prosser, changed his sheets and tended his wound. The whole time he spent apologising for inconveniencing us, ashamed of his wound and his smells. Mr Prosser always tried to disguise the pain he was in, but at times his tight, flinching face gave him away. His treatment by Dr Jerrams had been harsh to say the least, and I had seen a couple of nurses act impatiently with him over the last few days, too. He was such a humble, good-natured man, never wanting to make a fuss, and it seemed a gross injustice that he was likely to end his days here, in this chaotic and unlovely place.

Once Sam and I had finished cleaning him up, Mr Prosser looked spent, his eyes dull and glassy. Sam left to attend another patient and I stayed to tidy up his room. After a few minutes I heard a dull thudding noise. I turned and saw Mr Prosser hitting his head against the bedstead. He was clearly in unbearable pain. Tears glistened on his stubble and his throat emitted a wheezy rattle. 'I just want to die, please, God, let me die. LET ME DIE!'

And then, just for a moment, I lost it. There were no words to express it. Mr Prosser's state was so enfeebled and monstrous, so iniquitous and grim, that I felt myself well up, too. Grief and outrage surged over me on his behalf. It was unprofessional and unhelpful, but there it was. During my stint as a student nurse there were other emotionally charged moments, but this was the first and only time I publicly shed a tear. I doubt I would have lost it if Sam had been in the room. But this was a private moment, Mr Prosser being too caught up in the introspection of his own pain to notice me.

A moment later I pulled myself together and went over to comfort him. It was clear the poor man had no fight left in him: he'd led a good life, and now wanted out, yearned to join his beloved Maureen. Without her, there was no future for him, just pain and embarrassment, and it would have been patronising for me to suggest otherwise. I simply held his arm and tried to tell him not to worry. I think I've rarely felt so useless. Soon he fell asleep and I returned to the other patients.

'Pretty rough for Mr Prosser, huh,' said Sam, as we were writing notes at the end of the shift. 'I don't think he'll live long now. Forget his leg, it's his heart that's broken, poor man.'

'Broken heart?' I asked. 'Do you think there is such a thing?'

'Absolutely, sweetheart!' insisted Sam, thudding her fist against her chest for emphasis. 'I've seen it loads of times. It doesn't appear in medical books, but it's common. Health care assistants know better than doctors about certain conditions, and this is one of them.'

Sam explained that bereaved patients often went radically downhill after the death of a partner, especially in the first few months. They showed increases in blood pressure, pulse rate and changes in their clotting systems, making them more prone to heart attacks.

'Of course, many mourners get over it,' explained Sam, closing a patient's file. 'They go on to lead active lives. But others are destroyed. Mr Prosser's wife was his life. Now he just wants to join her. Pretty obvious, really. Don't need a doctor to tell us that.'

It was my last day with Sam, and I thanked her for looking out for me. Tomorrow would be my final shift. The ward had unquestionably been my worst to date* and I had often been worried for the patients. But it had also given me an insight into the challenges of adult nursing and, even in this short time, I knew it was not for me.

That night I did military fitness in the local park. I'd been going more regularly and was really starting to enjoy it. I remember that particular session as, on arrival, I was still very churned up about Mr Prosser. But once I'd changed into my sports kit, I did my best to forget about him. Normally during the warm-up run I would be stumbling along with the stragglers. That evening I was on fire and ended up in the leading posse. I wanted to feel

---

*The ward has since had a massive refurbishment, and, according to a nurse I know who works there, is much improved – now not only fully staffed but run by a top-class matron.

my heart pumping like fury, smell the mineral stink of the grass as we did our press-ups, my blood charged and vibrant. I wanted to try to forget Mr Prosser and his broken heart and, until the next shift, guiltily rejoice in my own blessed luck.

Chapter 9

GOING MENTAL

'Mate, please, spare me the details,' said Jake, leaning over the snooker table to pot a red. 'I'm squeamish about things like gangrene.'

It was the day after the Mr Prosser incident and I was telling Jake about it, clouding the facts to protect confidentiality. Over the last months I'd seen very little of Jake, and nothing of Bill, who'd recently moved to the country with his young family.

'I feel for the poor bloke, I really do,' said Jake. 'It must have been awful for him being treated like that. And that doctor sounds like a pillock. But don't let it get to you, Jimmy. You did what you could.'

Jake focused on his next shot. He wasn't proving the best person to reflect with about Mr Prosser. He was too absorbed in thrashing me at snooker. We'd had three games already and he'd won all of them.

Still, in many ways I didn't really want the advice. I'd just wanted the company of my oldest friend, especially now Jess was gone: someone outside of the hospital to have a drink with and enjoy some banter.

'We should do this more often, Jake,' I said. 'It's been weeks.'

'Yeah, sorry buddy.' Jake nodded while chalking his cue. 'I've been flat out. Some big changes going on.'

'Oh, really. What changes?'

Jake smashed the black ball into the far pocket and smiled at his victory. He could now focus fully on the conversation.

'I've been meaning to tell you, Jimmy.' He slapped me on the back. 'Anna and I are moving to Spain. She's got a posting in Madrid and I've lined up work at a language school there.'

'Madrid!'

'The fun of having a multi-culti relationship, amigo.' He shrugged. 'It's only fair I spend some time in Anna's country. She's been in England for five years. It's my turn now.'

'Wow, good luck to you. It must be love.'

'It is, Jimmy. She's my soulmate.'

'I can't believe it.'

'I know,' said Jake. 'If I'd have used the words 'soul' and 'mate' in any context a few years ago I'd have asked you to shoot me . . .'

'No, not that,' I interrupted. 'I mean first Bill becomes a commuter and buggers off to the sticks. Then I split with Jess and next thing, you hightail it off to Spain. You're all deserting me.'

'We're all settling down, Jimmy. Nesting up. You need to find yourself a nice girl to help iron your uniform and grow old with.'

'Tell me about it, señor,' I said. 'Until then I've got nursing to keep me on my toes.' I downed my pint and looked at my watch – 9 p.m. 'Shit, Jakey, got to dash. I'm on an early tomorrow. Good luck to you, you jammy bastard. Let me know when you're having a leaving party.'

We embraced. Over the last few months I'd lost Jess, Bill and now Jake. They were all moving in fresh directions – I was staying put. It felt like the end of an era.

My next placement was at a children's nursery. God only knows why.

At college we had been told that spending time among healthy children – as opposed to sick ones – would be invaluable as a means of comparison. To my mind the comparison was fairly obvious: sick kids – in bed, healthy kids – running around shouting. But no, we were told, we would discover what makes healthy kids tick, what interests them, how to calm them in a tantrum. We might even rediscover the joys of hopscotch and conkers. I had nothing against all this, but it did sound rather flaky.

It certainly turned out to be the easiest week of the course. But just because I had an easy time, doesn't mean nursery workers normally do. Keeping thirty children aged between two and five occupied all day is no mean feat. But it was OK for me, as, unlike at the hospital, all I really had to do was muck around.

Every day from 8 a.m. to 4 p.m. I spent my time playing football, playing draughts, playing What Time is it Mr Wolf? I read stories, caught leaves in the wind and sang nursery rhymes. I'm not sure how much I learnt, especially as I already have a daughter plus an army of nieces and nephews. Still, it was a nice break from the hospital.

Before I started at the nursery I was given a pep talk by Fred, the whiskery head teacher, a gentle, quietly efficient Mr Chips type – and the only male member of staff. He insisted I never spent time alone with any child. I had no problem with this – it applied to all new members of staff.

'It's not just about protecting the children,' said Fred, clearly uncomfortable with having to lecture me. 'It's also to protect you from any false accusations.' I had already been through a thorough CRB check, but now I was out of the hospital different rules applied. I had no axe to grind over this, it was common sense.

Over the next week I never once felt awkward being the only man at the nursery other than Fred. It seemed to me that the reason why there are so few male nursery workers* was down

*Currently more than a quarter of English state primary schools have no male teachers at all.

to the general climate of mistrust whipped up in the media over men working with young children. There's no question CRB checks on all nursery staff are essential, as are common-sense rules, but too much paranoia doesn't help matters.

What I remember most about the nursery, though, was the great staff – especially Maggie, a West Indian teacher of Amazonian stature with a rich, drawly voice. She called everyone 'darlin', and gave me the nickname 'posh Jimmy' as I liked Earl Grey tea and spoke with 'a bit of a nobby accent'. She was a whizz with the children, and always good at defusing any playground fracas. Several times throughout the day she would encourage the kids to sing along with her, whether to 'Baa Baa Black Sheep' or the latest hit by Take That.

By the end of the week I had developed a huge crush on her, and finally plucked up the courage to ask for her number. I knew very little about her, other than she was way out of my league, but there was still no harm in trying.

'Tell you what, Jimmy,' she said, once I'd spoken to her. 'You give me your number and let's take it from there.' This was clearly a polite way of telling me to get packing. But she was still kind enough to ask all the children to draw me a card as a leaving present.

Walking to the bus stop with Maggie after my final shift I asked her if she ever got fed up working with children – fed up with all the new, over-the-top rules.

'I've worked with kids all my life,' she told me. 'I've had more CRB checks than hot dinners. No problem with that, it goes with the territory. You just have to rise above it.' She smiled and shrugged her shoulders. 'It's got pretty silly lately. Parents not allowed to video their kids at nativity plays. Paranoia over which adults can do the school run. But this is a job I love and I'm not going to let anyone intimidate me out of it. Nor should you, Jimmy.'

I shook Maggie's hand before she jumped on her bus. Later that evening I opened the children's farewell card and punched the sky with delight. Maggie had written her number on the back of it, along with a message: 'Busy for a while, but feel free to call next month.'

Although I couldn't wait to call Maggie, it wasn't such a bad thing to hold on a while. I still had some big decisions to make, most pressingly whether to switch from children's nursing to another branch.

Recently we had been given a lecture by Tanya, a sixty-something ex-ward sister, with silver hair and a taste in loud jumpers. Tanya's lecture had focused on mental health nursing, and really struck a chord with me. The woman was a force of nature, as verbally eloquent as she was physically clumsy. Her lecture was delivered in an arm-waving torrent, so hungry was she to impart her information.

Tanya's lecture not only championed mental health nursing, but provided a brief history of mental illness. Due to time restraints she ping-ponged from subject to subject in a wildly erratic manner, but it was spellbinding stuff. She began by explaining that the word lunatic stems from *luna*, the Latin word for moon.

'In ancient times insanity was thought to be caused by too much water in the brain, my dears,' said Tanya, ruffling her long hair. 'The moon dictates the movement of the tides, so it was believed to be connected to madness. Now, let's move over to the Greeks . . . '

We learnt that it was the Greeks who first coined the word *hysteria*, meaning womb. Back in the time of Socrates it was believed the uterus could break free from its moorings and influence the body, as far up as the brain, leading to sexual disturbances and mentally unusual behaviour.

'All this was Before Christ,' stressed Tanya. 'There were no feminists around to challenge the logic.'

Tanya then dramatically leapfrogged to Britain in the late 1700s: a time when a few thousand 'lunatics' were housed in asylums – the numbers growing rapidly throughout the next century. It interested me to learn one definition of asylum stems from the Latin: *a* – without, *sylum* – cure, as if the patients at that time were beyond help. The word asylum in its more benign context – as a place of refuge – only came into play more recently.

'So if you think it's bad in the NHS now,' stated Tanya, wagging a finger at us all, 'think what it was like then, my dears. It was a time when some still believed human thought was generated in the stomach or heart, and not in the brain. How about that, hah!'

She explained that the asylums in England varied greatly in their levels of compassion. In certain places it was possible for the public to gawp at the patients. At the notorious Bethlem Hospital in London visitors were even permitted to bring long sticks to poke inmates, the more mentally unwell the better. A few 'mad doctors' dabbled with cures for insanity, but many were just too busy: in some asylums it was not unusual to have only one doctor for up to 500 patients.

The subject of mental health continued to be controversial into the next century, explained Tanya. She cited shell-shock victims from the First World War receiving electric shock treatment to 'cure' them so they could hurry back to the trenches. Things didn't improve much. During the 1940s and 1950s thousands of lobotomies* were conducted on patients deemed mentally

*Lobotomies were made illegal in the Soviet Union in 1950, where it was decided they turned 'an insane person into an idiot', but continued to be practised in America, the UK and some other parts of Europe for another decade. One high-profile person who underwent a lobotomy was Rose Kennedy, President John F Kennedy's younger sister. She was controversially lobotomised at the age of twenty-three in 1941, after bouts of mental illness, and lived in institutions until her death in 2005.

incurable, as was 'trepanning', in which a hole was drilled into the skull to relieve pressure beneath the surface. Lobotomies, increasingly viewed as barbaric, were almost wholly phased out by the 1960s in the UK, as other remedies, especially anti-depressant and anti-psychotic drugs, became available.

Tanya stressed that even now, with sophisticated brain scans, breakthroughs in medication and a much greater understanding of genetics, mental illness is a far from exact science. She accepted mental health was less stigmatised today, and its treatment more empathetic, but even so, whether dealing with depression, Alzheimer's or schizophrenia, there was still no precise cure.

'That's it on the history, my dears,' said Tanya. 'Over 2000 years of mental illness distilled into half an hour. Not bad, hey!'

'What about Freud and Jung and all of those clever people?' said Coco.

'Oh, don't get me started on Freud, dear.' Tanya put up her arms, as if in surrender. 'All that stuff about sex, the id and the ego, the Oedipus complex. Pah! It would take months. You have to switch to mental health nursing if you want to learn about that. Let me tell you a little about what it involves.'

Tanya told us that up to one in four people suffers from mental illness in their lifetime. She had worked in general nursing for years, but it was when she changed to mental health that she gained the most satisfaction. She had spent much of her time as a psychiatric nurse working on forensic wards. Murderers, rapists, paedophiles and other criminals were among her patients.

'Nothing tests your empathy more than nursing a man who has killed his own wife and daughter,' explained Tanya, standing unusually still. 'In some cases it's hard to forget the criminal and see the human being. But that is what you have to try to do. No physical wounds are visible with certain patients, so you must always strive to see the mental ones.

'The brain is not only my most vital organ,' added Tanya, while sketching a brain on the board. 'It's also my favourite organ, or, according to Woody Allen, his second favourite organ.' She rolled her eyes and laughed. 'Never forget, if our brain stems are severed we are dead.' She stabbed a finger at her diagram. 'Our brain is what keeps us alive, but most importantly our brain is what defines who we are, our personality, what makes us human.

'Today King Solomon is remembered for his wisdom,' concluded Tanya, tapping her forehead. 'But when asked by God what he most wanted, Solomon asked for "an understanding heart". I'm an atheist but I believe an understanding heart is the key to working in mental health.'

This lecture – which had crammed science, history, comedy and King Solomon into forty-five minutes – had been entirely different to all our other nursing lectures. I had often enjoyed classes to date, but after this one I was on a high – both excited and curious to learn more. I was surprised that none of the rest of the group felt the same way. In fact, Tanya's lecture seemed to have left many of them cold.

'But mental illness affects so many people,' I said at lunch in the hospital canteen. 'One in four of us at some point – that's massive. I think mental health nursing would be really rewarding.'

'No way I would do it,' said Jana, spearing a rubbery tube of pasta. 'All that verbal abuse, the constant threat of violence. I'd find it really tough. I want to stick to kids.'

'That's overstated,' I said. 'I'm sure only a few of the mentally ill are physically violent. And besides, you're bound to have good back-up teams. Alarms and all that.'

'It still sounds dangerous,' agreed Coco. 'And it's not like proper nursing, really. Something else altogether.'

I knew both these points were regular criticisms labelled at mental health, that it was one: dangerous, and two: a lazy, half-baked type of nursing that lacked the credibility of more hands-on work. But over the last year I thought of how many times I had brushed with mental illness on the wards. I thought of Sally's suicide attempt and Mr Smith's drink-related violence, of Julius's depression following his diagnosis of Crohn's disease, of Mr Prosser's gangrene and his resulting mental turmoil.

Then there was the personal impact. All of us know somebody with mental illness – maybe a parent with dementia, a friend with schizophrenia, a work colleague with depression, a cousin who self-harms, a daughter with anorexia, a spouse addicted to drugs or maybe just a neighbour who shouts to himself.

'Wouldn't you miss working with children though?' asked Vicky, as I continued to champion mental health.

'Maybe you could combine the two,' suggested Jana, while rolling up a cigarette, 'and work in children's mental health.'

'I suppose I could,' I said. 'But it's just a fleeting idea. I'll probably stay with you lot . . .'

'Thank God,' interrupted Vicky, pinning down my arm. 'I'm not sure I can stand losing another member of the group.'

But Tanya's lecture had sprouted a seed in my mind, and it would continue to grow over the ensuing weeks.

For my last placement of the year I wasn't to be cooped up in a ward or a nursery – I was going to be on the street. I was looking forward to it: I'd always fancied the outdoorsy, pavement-pounding element of community nursing.

My role in the community was with a team of health visitors – qualified nurses who specialise in promoting a specific area of health. My mentor was Jane, a genial, heavy-set Zimbabwean woman, who liked to wear necklaces with baubles the size of golf balls. Jane's work focused on advising mothers with young babies.

This was not my dream placement at all. Jane was a great

mentor, but babies were never my forte. All that compulsory cooing (ooh, so sweeeet!) and nappy changing – like a toxic-smelling form of origami – left me cold. Also, unlike the wards where I could make myself useful, with health visiting I was nothing more than Jane's shadow.

Aspects of the work were interesting, though, and often shattered my preconceived ideas.

I remember one gloomy, overcast morning Jane and I entered a tower block in one of the rougher parts of town. There was graffiti on the walls, rubbish strewn around the stairwell and a few needles, clearly used for shooting up, in the communal lift. I expected the worst for the baby we were visiting. But on arrival on the top floor of the block we were ushered into a little oasis of domesticity: a warm, tidy flat, full of family photographs and framed tapestries. Jaunty sitar music played in the background. Like so many tower blocks Jane and I visited, this one was grim from the outside, but amid all the squalor there were proud havens hidden within.

Many of Jane's visits were to Bengali households, where the birth of a son was deemed as life's ultimate treasure. This was one such household. Not only was there the joyous mother and father, both in their early twenties, but an elegantly dressed grand-mother and an aunt, who had recently flown in from Bangladesh. Joining the happy scrum around the cot was Famin, a teenage neighbour, sporting jeans and a tracksuit top. She peered down at the baby and kept repeating: 'He's so beautiful, innit.'

Famin, a Bengali who had spent most of her life in the UK, had come to help translate as none of the baby's family spoke English well. The young parents had moved to England only two years earlier. Jane later told me it was common for Bengali children to help with translating, as they often spoke far better English than their parents' generation.

The little flat was fit to burst but there was something so relaxed and comforting about it. Jane and I were offered tea and cake as if we were somewhere in the Home Counties, while Jane asked her usual questions – baby feeding OK? Sleeping OK? Family all coping? Famin said the baby and the family were fine. It was clear the little boy would be positively showered with love here, and soon we were on our way.

The next home we visited, though only half a mile from the tower block, seemed a different world. Outwardly, this was the sort of place you would expect a child growing up to want for nothing. The house was a semi-detached manse, with a mani-cured garden. Indeed the lawn looked so neat, it might have been shaved, and the flowerbeds were studded with rows of tulips.

At first all seemed fine. Jane chimed the bell, and, on hear-ing the security buzzer, pushed open the heavy, black door. We were welcomed by Jessica, a woman in her early forties with a nervous smile. Considering she had only recently given birth she looked surprisingly gaunt, with lank, mousy hair that spilled down her back.

Her baby daughter, Hannah, lay swaddled in a blanket on a spotless blue sofa. The house was very formal, full of ornate curtains, oil paintings and lush, springy carpets. Jessica, despite her outward confidence, seemed very alone in it.

She explained to Jane that her husband worked long hours as a financial consultant. She, too, was in business, but was now on maternity leave. Having a baby was a radical change of lifestyle for her and she was having trouble adjusting.

'I'd been so looking forward to having some time off,' said Jessica, peering anxiously down at her daughter. 'I thought it would be relaxing with Hannah.' She paused, her lip quivering. 'But it's so tough. So boring and draining. And I feel so alone.' She wiped away some tears. 'God, I sound like such a bitch. I love Hannah, but it's so hard. My job was easy in comparison. I knew exactly what to do.'

Jane put a hand on Jessica's knee, and smiled. This gesture caused Jessica to weep uncontrollably.

'Perhaps, you should tell your husband how difficult this all is for you,' suggested Jane softly.

'But I can't,' insisted Jessica, controlling her tears. 'He just wouldn't understand. He comes back late from work, and tells me I'm so lucky to be with Hannah all day. How can I tell him I'm miserable?' She reached out to her baby and tenderly touched her. 'When I can't get Hannah to breastfeed I cry hysterically. My husband would never understand. He's ecstatic he's a father. Wants to tell the whole world.'

Jessica was clearly very isolated. All her family lived miles away and the couple had few friends in the area due to their furiously busy lives. Jessica was permanently exhausted, something she blamed on being a first-time mother in her forties. When Jane asked about hiring a nanny to help, Jessica resumed her tears, admitting she and her husband were mortgaged up to the hilt.

Jane insisted on another meeting, next time with Jessica's husband present. By the time we left the house Jessica had calmed down, but she was still clearly very vulnerable.

As we walked back to the clinic, I reflected on our experiences at the two homes. On paper, my chief concern would have been for the young, blue-collar Bengali couple living in a tower block and unable to speak much English. Instead it was the professional mother on maternity leave, living in a desirable post code with a high-earning husband, who needed the support.

'Always keep an open mind in this job, Jimmy,' said Jane, as we tucked into sandwiches back at the clinic. 'It throws up surprises every day. That's why I love it.'

I could see why Jane loved her job, but it really wasn't for me. Shadowing her, day in day out, weighing babies, proffering advice on sleep times and breast feeding, soon became a drag. Rather than being a mute sidekick I wanted to play a more active role, and so joined up with the clinic's district nurse, Celia, who agreed to take me on her rounds for a couple of days.

Celia was a short, slender Nigerian woman whose fragile looks belied considerable stamina. She would zoom between patients' homes in her Smart car. One minute we would be checking the blood sugar of an elderly diabetic confined to his bedsit, the next monitoring the progress of a school headmistress felled by a kidney infection.

One of the visits with Celia, I will never forget. Before our arrival Celia had filled me in with some background. The patient was, bizarrely, Celia's old boss, a nursing sister called Trish, who was currently undergoing chemotherapy for breast cancer. A large lump had been located two months earlier, which fortunately hadn't spread to the lymph nodes. Since then Trish had received chemo every three weeks in an attempt to shrink the tumour.

We were led into Trish's bedroom by her daughter, Eli, a serene-looking girl with long, dark hair and a nose ring. She had taken a break from university, where she was studying law, to look after her mother.

The chemo had been making Trish feel wretched, and, normally an active soul, she now needed Eli to help her to do the simplest things – walking, dressing and eating. It was noon but Trish was still in bed. She smiled weakly when she saw Celia.

'What's that you've got on your head, Trish?' asked Celia, pointing at her in mock horror.

'Oh, it's a fez I bought in Morocco years ago,' said Trish quietly. 'Never worn it till now. Might as well look chic, even if my hair has fallen out.'

'You call that chic!' Celia rolled her eyes. 'You look like a bloody leprechaun.'

Eli laughed at Celia's joke and softly kissed her mother on the forehead. She announced it was time for her to make lunch and skipped past me towards the kitchen.

Celia and Trish clearly shared a good camaraderie and I left the room for Celia to carry out her observations, and for the two friends to talk in private.

I joined Eli in the kitchen, where she was already busy preparing Trish's lunch, a vegetarian dish with lots of carrots, garlic and broccoli. She jived her head in time to a Madonna song playing on the radio.

'This meal is mum's favourite,' she said, chopping up a clove of garlic. 'She's really changed her diet lately. She's cut out milk, cheese and meat, and is eating lots of vegetables.'

'How are you holding up?' I asked.

'I'm fine,' she said, smiling. 'This is where I want to be until mum's better. Then I'd like to go back to uni.'

I asked if there was anyone else in the family who could help out. Eli explained she was an only child. Her father was only fifty-five years old, but was suffering from a rare form of early onset dementia, which was like Alzheimer's, except it affected people under sixty-five. Only 1 per cent of dementia patients got it, Eli told me, so it was hard for her dad to get his head round it, especially as he was diagnosed when he was only forty-nine.

Eli stopped to add some spices to the saucepan. The smell of lunch now dominated the kitchen.

'I remember playing football with dad one day.' Eli kicked at an imaginary ball. 'But he just kept missing the ball. I knew something was up – he was usually brilliant. Mum started noticing stuff at home, too. He kept forgetting keys, losing his wallet. We couldn't believe it was dementia when we were told. At his age! Not even fifty! He had to give up his work as a dentist straight away.' She smiled sadly. 'He's larger than life my dad. His charisma's mostly drained away now. I'm just so grateful to have known him before all this. Know what a great dad he is.'

'Where is he now?'

Eli told me her father was in a nearby home. Her mother had cared for him before her cancer and Eli had come back every weekend from university to help out.

'Since mum's illness we just couldn't cope looking after dad too,' said Eli. 'I visit him most days now. It's sad though. He sometimes doesn't know who I am.' She frowned as she drained the vegetables. 'I hope we can bring him back here when mum's better.'

Eli was only nineteen years old, but appeared much older. I thought of myself at her age, and how distraught I would have been in her shoes: trapped at home, no social life, a father with dementia and a mother with cancer. She was young and bright and missing out on a key year at university. But rather than rage against her fate, she knew this is where she wanted to be. Sometimes working as a student nurse you meet people who not only impress you, but, through their own shining examples, really touch you, make you want to do better, to be better. Eli, though still a teenager, was such a person.

She was also very clued up. I learnt from her that in Europe at the time, only Estonia and Poland had worse cancer survival rates than the UK. Breast cancer survival rates though, she added, were much better than most, around 80 per cent, and she had no doubt her mum would recover.

'Mum is so lucky to have Celia,' said Eli, ladling the food on to a plate. I noticed Eli often used the word 'lucky'. 'Celia and mum go back a long, long way. There's a lot of respect between them. She's helped keep mum's mojo up, and isn't afraid to take the piss out of her.'

Eli put the lunch on a tray and carried it to her mother's bedroom, where Celia had just finished with Trish. We said our goodbyes. Celia seemed upbeat as we walked back to the car. She was pleased to have heard that Trish's latest test results had shown her lump had shrunk considerably.

'Trish has been through hell and back, poor love,' said Celia.

'But I've never heard her make a fuss. She's a great boss, a great nurse, too. Her husband was a friendly, active man, before his dementia. Now he's deteriorating fast. Trish was always there for him. It broke her heart to put him in a home, but she had no choice.'

'Eli seems pretty amazing, too,' I said.

'I don't believe in angels,' replied Celia, as we squeezed into her Smart car. 'But I think Eli is the closest I've ever got to meeting one.'

After my community placement I swore I would never weigh another baby in my life – but, to be fair, I'd learnt a lot working with Jane and Celia.

During the following fortnight I managed to pass my seven computer exams and finish the remainder of my nursing coursework. The foundation year was almost through.

Our last lecture of the year was by Mr Temple. He was friendlier these days, but even so, he was doom-mongering again that morning, telling us how tough the second year would be. 'You'll need all the help you can get!' he insisted. 'But I'm always here for you! All of you! Well, all except Jimmy!' He was right, he wouldn't be there for me. Having pondered for several weeks, I decided, at the eleventh hour, to swap from children's nursing to mental health.

Down in the pub that final evening, I was given stick for abandoning an already decimated group. We learned from Hadia that Shima was another casualty.

'She's homesick and a bit fed up,' Hadia told us, sipping on a coke. 'She might try nursing again in a few years when she's a bit older. She's found it all a bit much.'

'What a shame,' said Jana. 'I can understand why, though. But as for Jimmy leaving, that's just traitorous. It's just us girls now. We're in no-man's-land.'

'Leave it out!' I threw my hands in the air in protest. 'I'm keen to specialise in children's mental health, that's all. But I promise I'll stay in touch. How can I forget my girls?'

'We'll shun you,' said Vicky, punching my arm. 'Now that you're going mental!'

Vicky suggested a toast to all the students who had fallen by the wayside over the past year. We toasted Penny and Esme, Mayla, Chips, Ola, Sheena and Shima. How could we have lost so many? It seemed like yesterday I had been taking the Maths test with Elsa, trying on uniforms, practising blood pressures. Another children's nursing group that had started at the same time as us, bar a few early casualties, had stayed largely intact. And the adult nursing group had lost less than half its initial intake. Our little group seemed cursed – or 'special' as Vicky preferred to say.

We raised a few more toasts: 'Super Nurse! The Beards! Mr Temple! Florence Nightingale! Bruce Springsteen! The Queen!' I lost track after that. We were all euphoric that we'd completed the first year. Vicky, Jana, myself and a few adult nurses ended up in the dodgiest of nightclubs. I insisted I was far too old but they dragged me along anyway. The club played lots of 1970s and 1980s music. I couldn't believe it. I was in heaven. They even played a bit of Led Zeppelin, which got me pogoing like a drunk uncle at a wedding disco. I hadn't behaved this way since I was twenty-one.

I was too late for the night bus and I ended up crashing at the nursing halls on Jana's floor. I woke up early the next day with a crick neck and a sore head. Later on, Vicky, Jana and I all dived into a local greasy spoon. As we tucked into bacon sandwiches, Queen's 'Another One Bites the Dust' started playing on the radio. Ever since Mr Temple had mentioned it – along with 'Nellie the Elephant' – during the CPR lesson, it had become something of a class anthem. We all began to laugh.

I raised my coffee cup and in my best Mr Temple voice said: 'Eight down, four to go!'

Vicky raised her cup, too: 'Eight down, none to go. From now on, no one else is going to drop out of the course, whether children's or mental health. OK!' We raised our cups in agreement. Sadly, it wouldn't work out that way.

Chapter 10

WE ARE BROTHERS

From day one, it was clear with mental health nursing I would have to plunge in deep. No time for snorkelling around in the shallows. Especially when the opening lecture was called: 'Just Get Over It – We're All A Bit Mad.'

The lecture was given by a man known as The Doctor. He was surprisingly dapper – most lecturers are scruffs – and possessed a fringe so straight you could have taken a spirit level to it. He looked more like the manager of a provincial building society than a leading expert on the mechanics of the brain.

I knew no one in my group other than Kiko, the Senegalese ex-soldier I had met at the beginning of the course. He gave me a friendly wave and gestured for me to sit next to him.

'Let me introduce you to the others, my brother,' he stated, pointing at each of his class members like an auctioneer taking bids.

Unlike my children's nursing group, I was no longer the 'token bloke'. My new colleagues numbered exactly half men, half women, and the average age was much higher, too, somewhere around the mid-thirties. I was one of the few white faces, with most of the others coming from Africa, Ghana, Zimbabwe, Cameroon, Liberia and Nigeria. There was also Nicola – a sassy, raven-haired girl from Cardiff, her inseparable Russian friend Nina, and a Scouser called Joe. Although the others had all worked on mental health wards during the first year, they, like me, had been lectured mainly on general nursing. It was the second year when the nursing specialities – children's, mental health – really kicked in.

'Did you know,' said The Doctor quietly, tapping his pen on a table to gain our attention, 'that in this country mental health accounts for up to one third of all GP consultations?'

He shook his head despondently. 'And yet, there is still a huge stigma attached to mental illness. This should not be the case, and I would like to explain why.'

The Doctor began by telling us the 'well-known' story of Phineas Gage, a railway worker, who in 1848 had an accident that caused an iron bar to shoot through his brain. Despite being lucky to survive and appearing physically fine, this once well-balanced, capable and energetic worker soon became lazy, impatient and aggressive. Indeed, Phineas Gage's mind was so radically changed that his friends decided he was 'no longer Gage'.

'So,' mused The Doctor stroking his chin, 'do our brains make us who we are?' He looked around at us. 'Gage's personality had been transformed by the bar through his brain, but was he still Gage? Or were Gage's friends right? Had he changed into someone else?'

'His body was the same,' said Nina, in her smooth Russian accent. 'But his mind was different.'

The Doctor smiled and nodded approval before stating: 'Did you know, ladies and gentlemen, that our personality comes from the Greek word, persona?' No one answered as The Doctor continued striding up and down the classroom. 'Persona means mask,' he added. 'And all of us wear several different masks every day.'

'Isn't fame called "the mask that eats the face?"' said Zee, a gravel-voiced student at the back of the class.

'Indeed it is,' replied The Doctor. 'It implies your very character has been eaten into.' The Doctor splayed his fingers over his face. 'You don't know who you are any more or what mask to wear. Look at poor old Michael Jackson.' He sighed extravagantly: 'None of us human beings are simple creatures.'

We moved on through a host of other moral dilemmas. My favourite story centred on an American psychologist, David Rosenhan. The Doctor explained that in 1969 Rosenhan persuaded eight of his friends (three psychologists, a psychiatrist, a paediatrician, a housewife, a painter and a student) to undertake an experiment* to find out that, if by claiming to hear voices, they would be viewed as mentally ill.

Over the next three years Rosenhan's team of fake patients presented themselves at twelve different American hospitals. All of them told health care staff they had heard voices in their heads. Once admitted to hospital, they all said that they felt fine again and the voices had stopped. But this did not stop each of them from being held in wards for between eight to fifty-two days. In this time they were mostly diagnosed with schizophrenia and collectively administered – but did not swallow – over 2,000 pills.

'Rosenhan was shocked by his experiment on several counts,' said The Doctor, flattening his fringe. 'He was shocked that none of the doctors or nurses realised he and his friends were sane – not one realised they had faked the voices. And he was shocked how neglected he felt by the hospital staff once he was diagnosed as mentally ill.

'Can you guess who first realised he was sane?' The Doctor looked at us, waiting for an answer.

'One of the other patients?' suggested Nicola.

---

*Rosenhan published the findings of his experiment in the journal, *Science*, in 1973. It was titled: *On Being Sane in Insane Places*.

'Exactly right, young lady,' said The Doctor. 'It was the other patients, not the staff, who realised he was faking.'

'So maybe we really all are a bit mad!' exclaimed Kiko, laughing.

'I'm glad you said that, Kiko.' The Doctor picked up a pile of papers and began to pass them round. 'We certainly all have the capacity to become mentally ill, and should be empathetic to those who already are. As psychiatric nurses of the future it is part of your job to stop the stigma.'

Later that evening I read through The Doctor's notes from the lecture. The final page was titled: NEVER FORGET. He had written on it, with typical panache, some lines from Lewis Carroll's *Alice's Adventures in Wonderland*.

> *'In that direction,' the Cat said, waving its paw round, 'lives a Hatter: and in that direction,' waving the other paw, 'lives a March Hare. Visit either you like: they're both mad.'*
>
> *'But I don't want to go among mad people,' Alice remarked.*
>
> *'Oh, you can't help that,' said the Cat: 'we're all mad here. I'm mad. You're mad.'*
>
> *'How do you know I'm mad?' said Alice.*
>
> *'You must be,' said the Cat, 'or you wouldn't have come here.'*

My new group were a likeable bunch. The African posse were always high spirited and often brought in home-cooked foods – yams, curries, spiced meats – which filled the classroom with exotic smells. They insisted we all shared the food. 'Eat it up, my brother, eat it!' I was particularly fond of Kiko, with his indefatigable attitude and Zee, a one-time car salesman, who was the class joker.

I also spent time with Joe, the Scouser, who had quite a bit of experience volunteering in psychiatric wards, Nicola, the girl from Cardiff, who was hoping to become a psychologist, and Nina, the Russian, who already had a degree in anthropology.

Despite liking the group, the dynamic was very different to the previous year. Much of the student bonding occurs in that strange, perplexing first year, and I still often met up with Vicky and Jana, with whom I had built up a strong sense of trust.

We also had far more coursework to deal with in the second year – nine essays and a telephone directory-sized portfolio. Free time would be much harder to come by. I would have to cut back on military fitness and weekend high jinks.

A saving grace of mental health nursing was the quality of the lecturing. Sure, there were still some duff classes. One especially dire class focused on the potentially interesting subject of 'emotional intelligence'. Ironically, it was taught by a man who seemed to possess all the emotion of a statue and the intelligence of a pot plant. But this was the exception, and usually we were treated to the calm wisdom of The Doctor or the arm-waving passion of Tanya.

Time flew by and I was soon being primed for my first placement. It was to be on a forensic ward filled with mentally unwell rehab patients referred from prisons.

And so, one frozen October morning, I found myself sitting in the ward's white-walled waiting room beside a jungly yucca plant. I was not wearing my nurse's uniform – very few mental health nurses wear uniforms – but still sporting my JIMMY FRAZIER name badge. Outside it was hailing – bits of shattered sky playing tunes on the window. I braced myself for my first shift as a mental health nurse.

The first thing that struck me about the ward was the pool table. There it stood, slap bang in the middle of the room, opposite the nurses' station. I had been told we could sometimes play pool with patients, but I imagined in a games room, not the ward itself. That's good, I thought, great stimulation for the patients. Then I noticed all the security features: the air-locked main door, the impregnable windows, the red alarm buttons on the walls and the fact all the nurses had more keys than a small-town sheriff. Not so good.

We were being shown around by a heavily bearded middle-aged Zimbabwean nurse called Tony. He told us he had initially come to England a few years earlier to work as an English literature teacher in an inner-city school. He had lasted three months.

'In Zimbabwe teachers are treated like princes,' said Tony, pushing up his black-rimmed glasses. 'I couldn't believe the school I taught at here. The children all swore at me! I took up nursing soon after.' He smiled, as he led us into the kitchen area. 'I still get sworn at, but at least now it's by patients who can't help it.'

Tony demonstrated some of the kitchen equipment as he talked. He told us to permanently lock not only the kitchen, but all the doors on the ward, whether the drug store or laundry cupboard.

'The Russian writer, Dostoyevsky, claimed the key to happiness is never to use locks,' said Tony, locking the kitchen. 'He surely wouldn't have been very happy here.'

Tony often quoted writers and talked in proverbs. He told us that all mental health workers seek relief from their job in different ways – sport, faith, alcohol – but for him nothing hit the spot better than reading a classic novel: 'the best therapy in the world – especially those Russians!'

After a peek in the medication room, the filing office and the nurses' station Tony told me and Kiko – who was also on placement here – to wander around the ward, speak to patients and make ourselves useful.

'Shouldn't we read some of the patients' files first?' asked Kiko.

'No,' replied Tony, running a hand over his bald scalp. 'As it's your first day, it's better just to talk to the patients.' He gestured towards a rack of orange patient files. 'If you read all their stories first you will form too many pre-conceived ideas.

Between them, they've done some pretty rough stuff – murder, rape, abusing members of their own family.'

'OK, we get the picture,' Kiko said, grabbing my arm. 'Let's go and face the music, Jimmy.'

We both walked into the ward's central area. There were a couple of dog-eared posters on display – one advertising an upcoming pool tournament. It was 8 a.m. and still very quiet, just the cleaner wielding a broom. Most of the patients were yet to wake up. Finally, one of them appeared. He was a stocky, olive-skinned man of about sixty with a thatch of black hair swept back in a pony tail and a ragged moustache.

'Good morning,' I said, as he walked past.

He stopped abruptly, like a sentry guard, and looked me up and down. 'Good morning is it?' He had a distinctive accent, Italian sounding. 'So what's good about it, then?'

'Well, it's not that good, I suppose,' I said. 'The weather's a bit chilly still.' I was trying to be friendly, but ended up sounding like the Major from *Fawlty Towers*.

The pony-tailed patient walked straight up to me, locked me with his rheumy brown eyes and said: 'You are probably the ugliest bastard I've ever seen in my life.'

Oh, shit. What the hell had I done now? I'd managed to wind up my first patient just by saying hello. Don't panic, I told myself. I had been given an alarm attached to my belt, which I could pull at any time. But it would be a bit excessive to pull it now, wouldn't it? A bit like pulling an emergency parachute without waiting for the main one to open. He'd only called me ugly, for heaven's sake. Not exactly polite, though, was it? Perhaps I should ask him not to talk to me like that, thank you very much? Or would that sound a bit uptight and patronising?

'I said,' the patient moved his face closer to mine, 'that you are probably the ugliest bastard I've ever seen in my life.'

'Yes,' I replied, fear in my voice. 'A lot of people have said that.'

'Ha!' he shouted. He smiled, revealing his ruined dentistry. 'Ha bloody ha!' With that he marched off and sat at tables where we would soon serve breakfast.

It turned out the verbally abusive man was called Pablo. Tony said he was well known on the ward. He had been there for over a year, and in and out of institutions – prisons, hospitals – most of his adult life. Pablo often told new male student nurses that they were 'the ugliest' he'd ever seen and new female student nurses they were 'the most beautiful' just to rattle them.

'The poor man is very unwell,' said Tony. 'He likes to intimidate, but he's very unlikely to ever hurt you.'

I told Tony that I had been unsure how to deal with Pablo's aggression. Were there any tricks I should know?

'Just try to always be calm and empathetic,' said Tony, while tidying up the filing room. 'I watched you. You were fine. There are no definite answers in this job. A bit of experience will give you more confidence. We all de-escalate patients in our own ways.'

'Oh, OK. So just stay calm, and do what feels right.'

Tony slapped my back. 'Don't look so worried, Jimmy! It's not always easy, but you'll be fine.' He moved his arm in a snake-like movement. 'Just try to be as wise as a serpent.' His arms then changed to a flapping motion. 'And gentle as a dove!'

That morning I helped with the medication round, served breakfast and lunch, and spent much of my time talking with the patients. Some clearly did not want to interact, while others were raring to tell you their life stories, their hopes, fears and dreams. And if not those, at least which members of staff or fellow patients were pissing them off.

Although some of the twelve male patients on the ward were standoffish or abrupt, many were rather charming. At times throughout the shift, I forgot I was talking to people with a history of violence and abuse, and saw Tony's logic in keeping Kiko and me away from the patient files.

After the shift's final handover, Tony signed off my timesheet and told me I could read the files tomorrow.

'Just to warn you,' Tony pointed at the piles of paperwork. 'Tomorrow you must try to remember the person you met today. You may find in the files that the man you were joking with this afternoon is a sex offender. Whatever they have done, try to always see the human being.'

Tony was right. We should always try to see the human being, but at times it was hard after reading about them. One man I had met the day before, who I had particularly liked, turned out to have abused his own stepdaughter. Another of the more sanguine patients was a multiple rapist.

But in some ways, reading through the files also helped me to understand certain patterns of behaviour. I noticed *all* the men who had raped and abused women or children, had themselves been sexually abused, or else suffered miserably as a child through physical or mental abuse. Several of them also seemed genuinely full of remorse.

Among the dozen patients, some were repeat offenders while a few had committed only one crime – usually in a spontaneous fit of anger. Often the look and personality of the patient did not fit the crime.

The most striking of these was Mr Hans, an elderly man of Hungarian descent who, on discovering his wife's infidelity, had beaten her into a coma. Now, imprisoned on the ward, Mr Hans hobbled around in his tweed cap, looking barely capable of making it to breakfast, let alone hurting anyone. Unlike the other patients and their tragic histories, he'd seemingly had a happy childhood, a loving family, and, until the fatal discovery of his wife's affair, an idyllic marriage. In one crazed instance he had lost it all.

Mr Hans now cut a pathetic figure, full of tortured remorse, shuffling around as if on some tragic pilgrimage: his only reward, an antidepressant and mood-stabiliser cocktail at lunchtime. He rarely engaged with the staff or the other patients. The only times I spoke to him was over games of chess, which he seemed to enjoy, and usually won.

'I'm just waiting for death now,' Mr Hans said, in his thick, drawly accent. 'I'm a left-hander – a southpaw.' He bunched his left hand into a fist. 'This means I'm likely to die nine years earlier than a right-hander? Thank God! I smoke too much and eat rubbish just to speed it up.' He looked down at his watch. 'I've only got a couple of years left on this fucking earth, maximum.'

I assured Mr Hans that many left-handers didn't die earlier, that the facts were inconclusive. But he was insistent on his own imminent demise. He reminded me of Jack Nicholson in the film *About Schmidt*, in which the bored, ageing anti-hero watches the office clock, willing it to reach 5 p.m. His life had seemingly lost all meaning and was just a begrudging limp towards the final curtain.

Other patients used their remorse more constructively. One attended cooking lessons, another learnt guitar, and several enjoyed developing IT skills or working out at the gym. The one thing that united them all, other than the pool table, was the television. This took pride of place on a wall in the centre of the ward, forever blasting out pop videos. Tony told me it was brand new – the last TV had been smashed by a suicidal patient who had wanted to slash his wrists on the glass.

That weekend was Jake and Anna's leaving party. All the guests squeezed into their tiny flat, tucked into Anna's paella and toasted the Madrid-bound couple with tumblers of sangria.

Gone midnight, the only people left were Jake, Anna, Bill (who had been allowed the night off from family duties) and me. Anna kissed us all goodnight, and Jake opened some whisky.

'Buena suerte, Jakey Boy,' said Bill. 'To you and Anna – best of luck.' We all clanged our glasses.

'And to you, Bill,' I said. 'Congratulations on Ingrid expecting again. What's that, number four?'

'You big stud, Bill.' Jake toasted him. 'Good on you, O earth daddy, O potent one.' We all raised our glasses.

'And to you, Jimmy,' said Bill, slugging on his whisky. 'As you're such a girlfriend-free sad sack we'll have to toast you and all the loonies you work with.' Jake raised his glass. Once we had all downed our drinks there was a brief silence.

'Seriously, mate.' Bill gave me a concerned look. 'It must be scary sometimes, isn't it, doing what you do?'

'You wouldn't believe it,' I said, lapping up Bill's hysterical image of my work. 'Some of my patients make Hannibal Lecter look like a vegan. Every day I fear for my life.'

But the honest answer was that – except for Pablo's initial 'ugly bastard' insult – I hadn't been scared on the ward, and I'm the biggest wimp in town. Witnessing mental illness first-hand certainly upset me at times. I'd come back from the odd shift exasperated, angry and exhausted. But not scared. After all, I'd been in a ward full of expert staff with alarms. What had I to be scared about?

For the patients though, I sensed it was often scary. Mental illness by its very nature is scary, whether it causes anxiety, paranoia, dark moods, hearing voices or a host of other distressing symptoms. In the media, those diagnosed with schizophrenia are viewed as especially dangerous and often negatively depicted – 'Loner!' 'Psycho!' 'Sicko!'

In fact, schizophrenia sufferers – one in a hundred people – are of more danger to themselves than to anyone else: around 10 per cent of them commit suicide, and many more attempt it. You've much more chance of being killed by somebody who is drunk, or in a car accident or even by a bolt of lightning, than by somebody with schizophrenia. And yet the stigma goes on, with many patients more distressed by the shame of their mental illness than by its symptoms.

Once I'd explained this to Bill he softened his stance slightly, but still wasn't completely convinced.

'Don't you think some of them are just a bit lazy?' he said. 'Need to get a grip. Pull their socks up?'

'I used to,' I replied. 'But most patients on psychiatric wards can't just pull themselves together. It isn't all in their minds. Their illnesses have strong biological and personal links.'

'I'm not so sure,' said Bill. 'But, here's to you, mate.' He looked pensively into his drink. 'I sometimes think I'm half bloody mad, too, getting up at dawn every day to commute to a job where I stare at a computer for ten hours.'

'You think that's mad?' Jake raised his hand in protest. 'You should try teaching the subjunctive.'

For all the trials of my friends' jobs, I sensed they were both very good at what they did. My job was much more hazy. With people like Mr Hans and Pablo it was hard to know if nursing made any difference at all. None of the patients' diagnoses were clear cut. Their moods often changed, as did their medication. At best, I could only hope that by treating them with respect, something they'd often been denied outside the ward, we improved their lives just a little.

'So no regrets about going mental, Jimmy?' asked Jake.

'None at all, Jake.' I told him. 'And talking of going mental, you're about to go to a country where they fight bulls, drink sherry and throw tomatoes at each other. Now that's really loco.'

'Not as loco as me facing three toddlers and a pregnant wife with a hangover tomorrow.' Bill rubbed his head. 'I suppose madness is all relative.'

The fortnight after Jake and Anna's departure I spent every day on the ward. There were many things I came to like about it.

For a start, I had much more time to interact with the patients than I ever did on the child or adult wards.

I enjoyed the ward's lack of hierarchy, too. Psychologists, psychiatrists and social workers, rather than restricting themselves to half-hour appointments with patients, often mingled with them on the ward, and regularly asked the nurses' point of view.

A good way to gauge the attitude of a ward is the way the health care staff treat the cleaner. On this ward the cleaner, an exuberant Jamaican called Jack, was very much part of the team. He took pride in keeping the ward spick and span. Indeed, when situations got high octane Jack was a champion at calming down a distraught patient – or nurse, or, best of all, a therapist! On some other wards the cleaners had been more like shadows, whom nobody spoke to, and who, in turn, spoke to no one.

The ward had lots going for it other than the united staff. The fact it was light and clean and decorated with bright pictures was another bonus. But, for all this, there were axes to grind, too. My main axe was not specific to this ward, but mental health nursing generally – the paperwork! There, I've said it! The dreaded NHS P-word. If you are still reading now, I salute you. I will keep this short.

All nurses deal with a mass of paperwork, and, as a student nurse it is only right that you do your share – find out what you are letting yourself in for. You will deal with essays and portfolios but it's also vital to read key nursing policies. In the first year, the document that eclipses all others is the snappily titled: *The Nursing and Midwifery Code of Professional Conduct*. This is top banana in the X Factor of nursing policy – the one all trainees need to know. And rightly so, as it protects the public, by making qualified nurses accountable for their actions.

Now that I had entered the enigmatic realm of mental health, the paperwork seemed to have doubled overnight. I quickly needed to master the Mental Health Act (covering the rights of patients in mental health services) and the basics of sectioning.

On this ward the most relevant section was Section 47 – the transfer to hospital of a person serving a prison sentence. There were dozens of other sections – some lasting up to six months, others only six hours. Some sections allowed patients an instant appeal to a tribunal or to refuse their medication – others categorically didn't.

Then came risk assessments. These are a vital part of nursing. Whether on your patient's admission, discharge, or all the times in between, constant risk assessments need to be written up. They can vary from the 'no shit Sherlock' obvious, such as keeping a suicidal patient under constant observations, to the more subtle, such as allowing a challenging patient to join a martial arts class.

The paperwork was never-ending, not only the risk assessments but the care plans, which regularly updated the best course of action to improve a patient's life. Some of the form scribbling was, of course, essential. But to me – admittedly a wet-behind-the-ears greenhorn on his first mental health placement – some of it seemed hugely repetitive and so detailed as to be impenetrable.

As students, the main paperwork Kiko and I got to deal with were the daily notes on individual patients. Each shift we would be allocated two or three patients. We would note down what they ate and drank, whether or not they took their medication, what activities they got up to, whether they had expressed any concerns and how they behaved.

The patient I seemed to be allocated most was Pablo.

Since calling me 'the ugliest bastard' he'd ever seen, on my first day, Pablo had become a little bit more amiable – but not much. He was a complicated man, whose moods could swing radically. In some ways he seemed adrift of his moorings, living in a fragile and embittered world of his own.

He had been diagnosed with schizo-affective disorder, a loose combination of a mood disorder mixed with the symptoms of schizophrenia. He had suffered from this for a long time, since his early twenties. Pablo's illness manifested itself in long, dark moods, coupled with the hearing of anxiety-inducing voices, usually saying hateful things about him.

Pablo's major crime had been to try to push a woman under a train. Something he claimed voices had told him to do. He had luckily failed to hurt the woman, but had subsequently shown a startling lack of remorse. This lack of concern for others, coupled with suicide attempts and bouts of manic behaviour, including public nudity and verbal abuse, had kept him institutionalised for most of his adult life.

Pablo had a superior and often abrasive attitude towards others. At times I harshly (and wrongly) judged this as less to do with his illness, and more to his self-absorbed personality. Another patient I regularly worked with on the ward was a rapist, who was clearly overwhelmed with guilt, and determined to get his life back on track. Somehow I empathised much more with his plight, than the less criminal but wholly unrepentant Pablo.

But I really wanted to help Pablo. His life appeared to be a living hell, from which he derived no pleasure. He chain-smoked, and lived off very sugary tea and slices of white bread – never a hint of anything as decadent as jam – which he joylessly shoved in his mouth, as if merely stoking an engine.

Pablo was of Italian gypsy stock. He didn't get a good start in life, living hand to mouth in various parts of the Mediterranean. Despite boasting a sometimes romantic image, many gypsies are unemployed, illiterate and have nowhere to properly call home. A high percentage of Italian gypsy families lose at least one child, of which Pablo's family were no exception: his baby sister died when he was six. Soon after, Pablo's mother ran away from her husband, who was abusive, and took young Pablo to live with some cousins in south London. Pablo never talked much about his history: only that he had no feelings for his family, except his now-dead mother. He told me he had 'no one' and liked it that way.

He swaggered around the ward, chest jutting out, occasionally firing off abuse at staff members or fellow patients. Some days he wept in his room, calling out for his mother: 'Mamma, help me, mamma.' Other times he liked to smear mascara around his eyes, making him look like a despondent panda. None of the other patients teased him over this. Pablo had moments of high camp but was also a powder keg of incipient violence. For all his quirks, he was not somebody to be messed with. In any conversation he mentioned how he hated everyone – this patient, that nurse, this actor, that singer. To say anything positive seemed beyond him. Hope was a word that had long vanished from his lexicon.

Many combinations of medication had been tried on Pablo to alleviate his mental turmoil. He was currently on lithium, a mood stabiliser, and clozapine, an antipsychotic drug, which had temporarily stopped him hearing voices. The drugs were not without their side effects, the lithium causing his hands to shake, and the clozapine giving him constipation. He was also obese, another possible side effect of both drugs.

I longed to find something that might excite Pablo, spark some joy inside him. He wasn't bad at pool, but took no pleasure in winning. Chess bored him, as did reading. He occasionally watched a bit of television, but never seemed very engaged.

One evening I accompanied Pablo to a jamming session at a social centre within the forensic complex. A group of volunteer musicians played a short gig, mostly old pop hits, throughout which Pablo looked bored stiff. Then the band invited the patients to have a go with the instruments. Several of them picked up guitars or microphones to have a singalong. Pablo, to my astonishment, made a beeline for the drum kit. He sat down, smiled regally and proceeded to bash away like Keith Moon on amphetamines. For about twenty minutes, his drum sticks on fire, Pablo looked in heaven.

As we walked back to the ward, Pablo said: 'I quite enjoyed that.' I can't tell you how good it was to hear those words. Of course I asked him lots of questions: 'Why did he like drumming?' 'Did it spark any memories?' All of which he answered with a frustrating: 'Don't know.' But this didn't matter. Just for a moment Pablo had been happy. With mental health nursing, sometimes it's the little victories that count.

I was lucky to have Tony as my first mental health mentor. His calmness, wealth of experience and philosophical take on life made him good company. I noticed senior nurses of his age – fifty-somethings – either became worn down and exasperated, with withering reserves of patience, or developed a Zen-like ease in which very little rattled them.

When Tony was in charge of a shift, he was always a master at defusing potentially explosive situations. One of the chief problems on mental health wards, as I was to learn over the next months, was the lack of staff. A certain number of nurses were always needed at the ward. If staff numbers were low, it meant patients waited ages to be escorted out on leave, whether a cigarette break, a gym session or to visit a relative. These breaks from the ward were often the highlight of a patient's day, and if there was no nurse available to escort them, things could get messy.

When patients got angry, the more uptight nurses got angry too. This was a disastrous tactic that ended up in a prolonged verbal slagging match that unsettled everyone. Tony, however, would disarm fury with charm, and never once showed a flicker of frustration or fear. The fact he was well over six foot and nicknamed 'the boulder' – due to his physique – might have helped, too.

But Tony also made an effort with the patients. He'd find out what music and books they liked. He'd remember their birthdays, and ask about family members who were important to them. He'd give some of them nicknames such as Hustler Joe, or Honest Frank, but was careful never to show favouritism. To my mind, the respect he'd earned from the patients was all down to the respect he'd shown to them. Some of the more burnt-out nurses – mercifully few on this ward – treated certain patients as enemies, out to get them, rather than people they were there to care for.

On my last morning on the ward, while having a wrap-up session with Tony, I asked him how he'd managed to cope with twenty-odd years working in mental health.

'How do I cope?' he mused, rubbing his forehead. 'I cope, Jimmy, because I'm lucky. I've been blessed with a loving wife and four children. I have a life outside of here that brings me joy. But come in here with too much shit floating round your own head and you're in trouble. You'll take it out on the system, the other nurses, or worst of all, the patients.'

He flicked through my portfolio and signed off my timesheet with a flourish.

'Some advice, Jimmy,' he added. 'Never be a nurse that looks at the patients and thinks, lucky them. Living here, well fed, lounging round all day watching TV. Life of Riley. It's actually a miserable life. Boring, restricted, each dealing with their own demons.' He stopped and jokingly shook my shoulders. 'And don't believe all that rubbish about mentally ill people all being geniuses. Of course, some are bright, but the vast majority have lower than average IQs. All those Hollywood films, like *A Beautiful Mind*, have a lot to answer for.'

'Don't you ever get angry, though?' I asked. 'Don't certain patients get to you?'

'Oh sure, Jimmy, but you should never show it. The way I see it, these patients, however crazy, violent or self-absorbed, are my brothers, just as much as the other nurses. We are simply lucky enough to be in a position to help.' He paused for a long time, staring down, as if puzzling over a chess move. 'You ever read *War and Peace*, young man?'

'Er, no . . . one of those books I've always meant to.'

'Well, you should read it.' He waved his finger at me. 'I was lucky enough to work as a lifeguard one summer while I was still a student in Africa. It wasn't a busy pool and I read lots of Russian novels. Phew, man, I learnt some wise shit from those. One scene from *War and Peace* really changed the way I thought.' Tony settled back in his chair, frowning in an effort to remember.

'Prince Andrey,' he suddenly began to narrate, 'is one of the book's heroes. He is wounded in battle and is lying in a field hospital recovering. He hears a scream, looks over and sees his arch-enemy, forget his name now, being carried in, mortally wounded. This enemy is a bad man, a drunken playboy, and Prince Andrey's rival for the girl he loves.' Tony wheeled his chair towards me, swept up in his story telling. 'Prince Andrey has always hated this man, but now he looks across and all he feels is love. Love for this frail, wretched creature. And all because his one-time enemy is a fellow human being, crying out in pain, near to death. All the hatred, the past bitterness, falls away, and only the humanity remains.'

There was a pause as I was unsure if Tony had finished.

'Great story,' I said, nodding. 'But what's it got to do with nursing?'

'Can't you see, brother!' Tony said, losing his usual calm. 'I think Tolstoy's saying we humans are all in this together: that we should try to accept everyone, whoever they are, whatever their faults. In some cultures those people like Pablo, who hear voices, are not seen as suffering from schizophrenia, but are revered as shamans or sages. In the bible many of the old prophets heard voices in their heads, and were respected as men of God.'

'But they were mostly positive voices,' I said. 'Not telling them hateful stuff. Not telling them to push women under trains.'

'Sure,' replied Tony. 'But do you see my point? In many ways I think madness, especially with an illness like schizophrenia, is the price we pay for being human. The price we pay for our gift of complex spoken language. Animals don't go mad like us. Maybe furious or rabid, but not mentally ill, hearing voices . . . '

'Are you saying animals are too stupid to go mad?'

'No, Jimmy, not at all,' stated Tony, appalled at my suggestion. 'Animals are smarter than us in many ways. Did you know that during that terrible tsunami in Sri Lanka hardly any animal corpses were found? Barely even a rat. That's because, unlike us humans, they'd all had some sort of sixth sense about the incoming waves and had fled to higher ground. A few elephants had even broken off their chains, knowing they had to get away.'

Tony stopped and looked me hard in the eye. 'But humans have one thing animals don't appear to – conscious thought, introspection, self-awareness. To be human, is to be vulnerable to madness.' With this Tony let out a whoop of laughter and slapped his hand on his thigh. 'Ah, Jimmy, I've talked too much. Way too much! If you remember one thing from me, remember your own luck.' He handed me back my portfolio. 'Remember if you are ever scared or angered or disgusted by a patient that very little separates you from them. Only that you are in a position to help. Remember that we are brothers, all in this together.'

Chapter 11

HARD KNOCKS, SOFT TOUCHES

For my next placement I was put on another forensic ward, this time a PICU – or Psychiatric Intensive Care Unit. The name PICU fills a student with equal amounts of excitement and dread. It's likely to be one of the tougher placements, full of mentally vulnerable patients who have been transferred – from prison, off the street, or other wards unable to cope with them. For all my external bravado I was bricking it.

As with many PICUs there were only a few patients – in this case seven – due to the intense levels of care each of them required. All the patients were male. Due to the potential for 'things to kick off' there was a padded seclusion room, used if ever a patient became too much of a risk.

PICUs tend to be pretty spartan places. This one had the obligatory TV and a poky yard at the back where patients could smoke or kick a football around. There was no pool table and no board games. A few newspapers were available to read, each having been carefully vetted to make sure none of the patients – some of them headline-worthy criminals – appeared in any of them.

The nurses here clearly liked this style of work. They were unflappable, thick-skinned types, who, I sensed, enjoyed the slightly edgy environment. My mentor was a rangy, soft-spoken nurse from Ghana called Obi. Being a senior nurse he was often busy and I spent much of my time with my second mentor, Sally, a delicate-looking blond woman in her late twenties.

My initial fear of the PICU evaporated within the first week. Sure, there were incidents of verbal abuse, and at one stage a rapid response team – staff trained in restraining patients – were called in to help with a newly admitted man who was threatening to 'kill all the nurses', but he soon calmed down.

In fact, much of the time the ward was a picture of serenity. But, as Sally warned me, when things kicked off on a PICU, all hell broke loose. I was about to find this out, but not before meeting up with my old nemesis, Mr Temple.

On my second Monday at the PICU I had to return to college for a lecture. It proved to be a lecture with a difference. For starters what were Jana, Vicky, Hadia and Coco doing among us 'mentalists', as Kiko sometimes called us? And then I heard a familiar voice.

'Hello, Jimmy Frazier.' Oh no, it could only be one man. 'So the student who jumped ship returns to us.' I looked towards the whiteboard. Mr Temple was gleaming at me. 'We're mixing the children's and mental health groups together for this session. And I'm in charge. Grand idea, hey, Jimmy?'

The next hour was a nightmare. Mr Temple treated the surviving children's nurses as his little darlings and mental health nurses as new prey, ready to terrify and humiliate. As I was a children's branch defector, I was his principal whipping boy.

'You look hungover, Jimmy,' Mr Temple said, as an opening shot. 'As you get older hangovers get worse, you know. You have less water in your body. You start drying up. Dehydrate in no time!' He smiled, piously. 'Personally, I don't drink at all.' I'm sure you don't, I thought, except the blood of new students.

Mr Temple held up a newspaper headline: BINGE DRINKING — THE RISE OF THE LADETTES. Just the sort of sensational story he would love. He often started classes with something he had read in the morning paper.

'Why is it that our young girls are drinking so much?' he asked.

'Twenty-four-hour opening times,' said Vicky. 'And cheap booze in supermarkets.'

'And what does the alcohol do to their bodies?'

'Girls' testosterone levels are boosted when they binge drink,' chipped in Jana. 'That's why they act all wild and laddish. Unlike men, their systems aren't used to the rush of testosterone.'

'Very good, Jana,' gushed Mr Temple. 'Though I'm sure you'd never act in such a way.'

'Oh no, never, Mr Temple,' Jana chirped, smiling up at him angelically. Bloody children's nurses.

'So,' said Mr Temple, scowling as he surveyed the mental health students. 'Binge drinking is just one thing affecting today's youth. But let's dig deeper. Today I want to talk about depression. Why are Britain's children some of the most unhappy in Europe?'

'Depression is all because of poverty,' shouted out Kiko.

'Oh really, Kenko!' snapped Mr Temple. He was never very good on names. 'So why are some stockbrockers more prone to depression than the average person? And why do lottery winners sometimes kill themselves?'

You had to hand it to Mr Temple, he could do put-downs faster than the Sundance Kid.

'Well, obviously not all depressed people are poor . . .'

'But that's what you said, Kenko,' interrupted Mr Temple.

'Yes, but . . . there's happy stockbrockers too . . .'

Mr Temple raised his hand, and Kiko's comments dissolved,

as fast as foam on a river. He'd been Templed. I knew the feeling only too well.

'Right, then,' Mr Temple stated. 'Who here has contemplated suicide? Wanted to do themselves in? Come on, hands up!'

'Only since the start of this lecture,' whispered Kiko.

There was silence, not a hand flinched. Did Mr Temple seriously think anyone would admit suicidal thoughts to him, a man who often demonstrated all the empathy of a rattlesnake?

'Well, I've contemplated suicide,' stated Mr Temple. 'And not just after reading one of Jimmy's essays.' He paused, eyeing us all.

'Really?' asked Joe, the Scouser, breaking the stunned silence. 'You've thought of killing yourself?'

'Yes, really, young man,' replied Mr Temple, stone faced. 'I have certainly thought of suicide, as have most people if we're honest. Never tried it, of course. But come on. I bet some of you have at least considered it.'

It was an interesting point. I suppose in my very darkest hours it might have flitted into my mind, but I'd certainly never got to the stage of writing notes or loading a shotgun.

'Well, it's clear some of you are lying,' said Mr Temple. 'Except perhaps the Afro-Caribbeans among you. Your suicide rates are far less. Suicide is often very frowned on in Africa. In fact, some African societies do not even have a word for depression.'

'Is that good?' asked Kiko.

'Good in some ways,' said Mr Temple. But not when people with serious depression are unable to talk about it. Or unable to take the right medication.

'But in the West we have become obsessed with staying happy,' Mr Temple added, as he walked between our desks. 'We think we need to be happy twenty-four seven. We forget that being human means being sad sometimes, too.'

'Or being bloody miserable in his case,' Kiko mumbled to me.

'Doctors are starting to give out antidepressants like Smarties, you see.' Mr Temple was on a roll now. For all his terrifying qualities, I'd forgotten what a great lecturer he was. 'Thousands of children, some as young as eight, are now legally given Prozac. It's prescribed so much in the UK that trace quantities have been found in drinking water. That can't be good.'

Mr Temple explained that there was a big difference between 'depression' – feeling sad over a short period – as compared to 'clinical depression' – a serious mood disorder that, at its most extreme, can lead to psychosis, self neglect or even suicide.

'I think it's hugely unlikely children are clinically depressed before puberty,' he explained. 'To me they are simply unhappy, moody. No need for pills.' He clapped his hands for attention.

'OK, people!' Mr Temple glared at us. 'Enough of this. Let's liven things up. How about a little exercise. I want all of us to think what it's like to be clinically depressed.' With his arms, he motioned for us to split into two groups. 'Get lively, people!' I joined my mental health colleagues while Jana, Vicky and co all split off with the children's branch.

Mr Temple clapped again. 'OK. The exercise! Very easy. I want you to sit with a partner and talk to them about something that makes you happy.'

I sat with Kiko and talked about Poppin. Kiko talked about beer. It was all very upbeat and animated with lots of eye contact. Mr Temple then told us to do it again, but for the other person to stop listening. With Kiko sitting ignoring me – scratching his nose, texting – rather than firing questions or showing interest, I soon waxed far less lyrically about Poppin's many talents, and Kiko's amber nectar lost its fizz when I ignored him, too.

'So, people,' stated Mr Temple. 'The moral of the story is to listen. Just listen. Children's nurses are usually very good listeners. What about your mental health lot? Any good, Jimmy?'

'I think you're a big tease, Mr T,' I replied. I didn't really say it. I just sat there trying to look menacing so he wouldn't ask me again.

'Any good, Jimmy?' he repeated.

'Very good, Mr Temple.'

Mr Temple walked over to the whiteboard and drew a picture of a sad face.

'With clinical depression,' said Mr Temple, 'it can feel like no one is on your side, no one wants to listen to you. Your life loses meaning. The future seems hopeless. But for them, remember it's the whole time – every day, every hour – not just when their mate has stopped listening to them.

'So, children's nurses!' Mr Temple smiled at his chosen few. 'Don't write off your mental health colleagues as no-good wasters. Well, except Jimmy. Realise what a vital role they play.' He swung his bald head, slow and lethal as a tank turret, towards our group. 'And mental health nurses, of course, you already know how lovely children's nurses are. But remember to always consider not only a child's physical health, but his mental health, too.'

Mr Temple closed his eyes and let out a deep breath. A few students pushed back their chairs and made to leave. He had already overshot by ten minutes, but, as always with his lectures, the time had flown. Kiko stood up to go.

'Wait, young sir!' Mr Temple pointed an accusatory finger at him. 'Naughty fellow. Just one more minute of your time, please.' He pointed at the board.

'The World Health Organisation,' said Mr Temple imperiously, 'states that depression is the fourth most important health problem in the world today.' He paused for effect and stabbed his finger at the board. 'But by 2020 it predicts that it will be the number one problem in the world.'

He stopped and scanned the mental health nurses. 'You lot better step up to the challenge.' He waved a hand at the door. 'Now go, before Jimmy changes his mind and deserts you to come back to us children's nurses.'

'We won't take him now, Mr Temple,' said Jana, winking at me. 'He's yours, all yours.'

The following day on the PICU, as Sally warned it might, all hell broke loose. The patient concerned was thirty-year-old Jacko, an intense, wiry-limbed man from Sierra Leone with John Lennon glasses and a thatch of short dreadlocks. There are some patients you are destined never to forget – for me, Jacko was to be one of them.

Jacko's family had suffered during Sierra Leone's long civil war and had relocated to London in the late 1990s. From the start Jacko, then in his early twenties, found it hard to acclimatise. Coupled with the wartime horrors he had seen – his father had been hacked to death by rampaging soldiers – he found South London's grey skies and small horizons depressing.

Jacko secured the only job he could find – in a biscuit factory in the Midlands – which took him away from his mother and sister. He worked long hours for meagre pay, with very little social interaction. In his spare time he smoked cannabis in his dingy rented room. Within a few months he became increasingly downcast, and started to hear disturbing voices in his head.

One Sunday Jacko threatened two women with a knife in broad daylight for no discernible reason. Fortunately, both of them escaped and neither was hurt. Jacko was imprisoned, where his mental state worsened. He continued to hear voices and got into several fights, before being transferred to a psychiatric ward.

He had been in different forensic units ever since.

Jacko could be tricky but there was something very likeable about him. He challenged the nurses about his medication and sometimes 'cheeked it' – hid the pills in his cheek rather than swallowing them. This took some cunning, as nurses regularly asked him to open his mouth to check. He enjoyed dancing to music on his stereo, practising karate moves in his bedroom, flirting with the few female nurses and chain-smoking roll-ups. When he was in a good mood, he was full of fun and jokes. He generated great warmth. But when the voices came back, often as a result of him skipping his medication, he could be hard to handle. One of the symptoms, likely to be post-traumatic stress from his wartime experiences, involved him dodging imaginary missiles. As funny as this behaviour looked, it was clear from the terror on Jacko's face that it was no laughing matter. He was full of fear: a deep-rooted, paralysing terror.

What was touching about Jacko was the relationship he had with his mother, who had stood by him since the start of his illness. Mrs J, as we all affectionately called her, was a small, cheerful woman with wonky glasses and a greying Afro perm. Mrs J was the best person to calm Jacko, to bring him back from the brink. But when Jacko needed to lash out, she would also be his principal target.

Indeed, one of the triggers for Jacko descending into psychosis – a generic term for a loss of contact with reality – was him making abusive phone calls to his mother. The language he used was some of the ugliest I'd ever heard. It wasn't the sort of thing you'd want to inflict on your worst enemy, let alone your loving, septuagenarian mum. Such is the cruelty of psychosis and the hallucinations and delusions it can stir.

The day after Mr Temple's lecture Jacko's behaviour had become increasingly erratic. That morning he'd started talking to himself, diving under tables, snapping at staff, and, most worrying, making horrible calls to his mother on the ward phone.

After lunch things kicked off big time, as they so often did, over a relatively trivial incident. One of the patients, Sid, a tall, languorous Glaswegian, had picked up a newspaper that Jacko had been reading. Jacko lashed out. Within seconds a group of nurses stood between Jacko and Sid. Jacko was in a state of full-blown psychosis. He was shouting things that were impossible to understand, interspersed with swear words.

Sally was in the middle of it all, trying to de-escalate Jacko. You couldn't help but admire her. She was almost a foot shorter than him, even with her frizz of blond hair. She was showing great pluck, giving Jacko calm but firm instructions. I stood by her side, my adrenaline levels off the scale. Then Jacko lunged out at Sid, a wild haymaker of a punch, quickly intercepted by Hugh the Screw, an ex-prison officer, recently recruited to the ward.

Instinctively I grabbed hold of one of Jacko's arms – the one he wasn't lashing out with. My heart pumped furiously, and I felt a surge of strength. But Jacko's power was overwhelming. Even Hugh the Screw, who was holding Jacko's other arm, was straining hard, the veins on his forehead pulsing.

After that, it was a bit of a blur. When restraining a patient, at least four trained staff are needed, one for each arm, one for the legs and one for the head. Someone should also check that the patient's airway remains clear. Between us we had it just about under control.

Soon the rapid response team had arrived, and another nurse, far bigger than me, took over. Obi, who had been holding on to Jacko's legs, looked up and shouted at me, 'Get away, Jimmy, you should not be here. You know nothing about restraint. Go! Check on the other patients.' He was furious, and rightly so. Students are not supposed to play any part in restraint, but to stand there gawping while others were piling in had felt wrong.

A doctor arrived soon after and insisted Jacko needed sedation. He was still screaming out and fighting wildly against those holding him. Obeying protocol Obi asked Jacko if he would mind taking some oral medication, but he fired back more abuse. Sally prepared a Clopixol-Acuphase injection, a quick-acting sedative but also an effective antipsychotic.

After Sally jabbed him, Jacko continued hurling abuse for a while before he began to quieten. When he was sufficiently calm he was led through the ward into the seclusion room.

A seclusion room sounds all very *One Flew Over the Cuckoo's Nest*, but it is there to act as a therapeutic environment for a patient who is either a risk to themselves or others: Jacko to a T. Once inside, Jacko was observed non-stop, with regular drinks and meals being offered. He was given special rubber cutlery and polystyrene plates to prevent him self-harming. And there were other rules, such as keeping his tea sufficiently cool in case he chose to throw it at someone. On top of this he needed regular physical observations – pulse, blood pressure – to make sure his sedative had no adverse effects.

Every time anyone entered Jacko's seclusion room – even just to give him a drink – at least four trained staff needed to attend. Seclusion is very staff intensive. Jacko's seclusion had taken place early into my shift. That day I was on a long shift – meaning twelve hours, instead of the usual seven and a half – and for most of it Jacko remained relaxed. As I had no restraint skills, I simply prepared his food and drinks, or tended to the other patients.

About an hour before I was due to go home, Jacko started becoming anxious again. I was talking to Sally when Jacko shouted at her to get him a cigarette. She politely told him this was not possible. Within seconds he started charging at the door, yelling bestially, and bashing his head against the wall.

Sally tried to calm him with gentle words, but he was out of control. He started to leap up, performing martial-art kicks against the reinforced glass panel. And then: *whump*! He vanished from sight, collapsing directly underneath the observation window. We could still hear him, though, crying out in distress. Sally called the rapid response team and soon four staff rushed in.

I watched from the observation window. Jacko was bleeding

from a cut on his forehead, but he was clutching his heel. 'It's his knee,' said Obi. 'Looks like he's shattered it. We'll need to get him to A & E.'

While some of the nurses prepared Jacko for his A & E visit, I served the patients dinner. Rather than ask questions about Jacko, they were all strangely subdued. I could understand this. Restraint is a grim and undignified process. Seclusion, too. Witnessing Jacko's treatment was a stark reminder of their lack of freedom and autonomy. Rather than kicking off, many of them seemed pensive, wanting to lie low.

The patients collectively looked up as Jacko was rushed through the ward in a wheelchair en route to A & E. Soon they were focusing on their meals again. Like Trappist monks disturbed by a fleeting noise they resumed eating in silence.

Jacko came back the following morning. He was impossible to recognise from the snarling, uncompromising man of the day before. He had switched back to his breezy, diamond geezer self.

'All right, Jimmy,' he said, as he was ferried into the ward. 'Sorry about yesterday. Don't know what came over me. I'm such a bloody nightmare, aren't I?'

Jacko did the rounds, making his peace with all the staff, then whizzed up the ward corridor in his wheelchair trying to perfect a wheelie. He was in the best of moods.

'I asked for crutches at the hospital, Jimmy,' said Jacko, skidding to a halt beside me. 'But I was told a wheelchair is better. They think I'm going to go psycho and use my crutches as a weapon. I suppose after yesterday they've got a point.' He waved an imaginary crutch at me and smiled. 'Ahh, Jimmy, why am I such a fuck-up, eh?'

Mid-morning the tai chi instructor arrived. Tai chi was one class Jacko never liked to miss. The instructor, Billy, was what you would imagine a tai chi instructor to look like. In a room full of a thousand people he would stand out a mile as the martial arts guru. Not only was he half Chinese, wiry and incredibly cool, but he was dressed in black pyjamas. He spoke in a slow, deliberate and poetic manner.

That morning he kicked off the class in typically enigmatic style.

'Don't be afraid not to follow the herd,' Billy said softly, adjusting his bandanna. And then added: 'Because where the herd's gone, the food's already been eaten.'

'Who said that?' asked Jacko. 'Bruce Lee? Confucius?'

'No, Jacko, it was Bob Dylan. Dylan is far wiser than Confucius.'

'I'm more of a Barry White man, myself,' said Jacko, hooting with laughter. He really did seem in the best of moods.

The tai chi class normally attracted only two or three patients, and one member of staff always joined in. Today, I volunteered. Jacko, who was watching the class from the sidelines in his wheelchair, begged to be included. His knee had been heavily bandaged, as had his head, but there was no reining him in. He expertly hopped up on his good leg, as smooth as a flamingo, and balanced against a nearby table.

'Good work, Jacko,' said Billy. 'Let's see how you get on, but if you're ever getting wobbly just stop, OK?'

Billy started breathing deeply, and we all followed suit. We were supposed to close our eyes but I kept mine open to check on Jacko. He seemed lost in the moment, absorbed in the rise and fall of his diaphragm.

'Now we will do our first move – hold the ball,' instructed Billy, moving his hands as if holding an invisible ball. 'Next up. Parting the wild horse's mane. Careful, Jacko.'

We began to slowly move our hands in unison but the spell was broken when Mrs J appeared. She was dressed in a bright purple shawl, her Afro perm bobbing as if alive, huge and brilliantined. On seeing Jacko she lit up with a smile and shuffled towards him. 'My boy,' she said, as the pair embraced. 'My lovely boy.' Jacko towered over her and pulled her head into his chest. Taking Billy's lead, the rest of the class stepped back respectfully.

'Hi, Mum.' Jacko's eyes welled up. 'I'm so sorry, mum. So sorry. All those things I said to you.' His words were coming out in a torrent. 'I love you, Mum, more than anyone in the world. You know that, don't you, Mum?'

'I know, Jacko, I know.' Mrs J patted his back and released herself. She stood back and looked Jacko up and down. 'What a handsome boy you are, dear!' She then resumed her hug.

'I hate this illness, Mum,' Jacko said, clutching on to his mother, as if the ground might open up beneath him and she alone could stop him. 'Hate the things it makes me do. Makes me say.'

'I know, dear. It won't stop me caring for you, though. You know that don't you?' She patted his cheek. 'Not when I know what a good man you really are.'

I thought back to a couple of days before when Jacko had been calling his mother the most unspeakable things, ranting at her, threatening violence. I thought of how many times this splendid lady must have had to deal with this over the years and how she had always stood firm, never faltered, a reservoir of unconditional love.

None of the other patients on the ward had anybody like Mrs J – visiting regularly, withstanding abuse with stoicism, not a single harsh word for her charming but tempestuous son. I was convinced it was through his mother's love that Jacko was able to retain his warmth and humour amid the torment of his mental illness and his bouts of vainglorious wrath.

After their embrace Jacko, pressing his palms together, bowed towards Billy and excused himself from the class. Obi escorted him and Mrs J to one of the meeting rooms to spend some time together.

After half an hour of parting the wild horse's mane and other such moves Billy told me to make some refreshments using his

special pot for green tea. Soon we were all sitting cross leg-
ged in a circle – Billy, three patients and myself – listening to
some of Billy's music. It sounded like a couple of whales mating
accompanied by a flute. On psychiatric wards you sometimes
find yourself in the most surprising situations.

Later in the day I reflected with Obi about the whole restraint
episode. Reflection is a huge part of being a trainee nurse. In
class we had been taught endless models on how to reflect – the
Gibbs model, the Driscoll method – but to my mind reflection is
a very personal process. Sometimes I needed to reflect with my
mentor, sometimes with a colleague and sometimes I just needed
to reflect by myself when cycling home after work. Reflection
varied from deep analysis, to a scratch of the surface, to forget
about it. Over the Jacko situation I was happy to take time to
reflect with Obi.

'So did you enjoy the restraint episode?' Obi asked me, leaning back on his office chair.

It was an interesting question, and apparently one he asked
every student after they had witnessed a restraint. I told Obi
that it was useful to have seen it, and yes, it had given me an
adrenaline buzz, but that no, I had hated it. In fact, despite the
professionalism by which it had been handled, Jacko's restraint
and subsequent seclusion had been grim.

'Good,' said Obi. 'If you'd enjoyed it you would be in the
wrong job. No nurse should enjoy restraint. The minute you get
a kick out of it, well, that spells trouble.' Obi tossed his pen in
the air and caught it. 'Restraint is all about keeping the patient
safe, and those around him. That's it. It's not a punishment or a
power kick.

'So what did you learn from it all?' asked Obi, watching me
carefully.

At the time, I gave him some pat answer about how I'd learnt
it was important so stay calm. In fact, I'd learnt something far

more important by simply watching Mrs J. Here was someone who had not only coped with her husband's brutal death and upheaval from her homeland but had been abused by her mentally unwell son, both physically (rarely) and verbally (often), over many years. Mental health nurses spend hours with the Jackos of this world, but there are lots of us, we have alarms, sedative medication, and if it all gets too much we can quit, walk away.

In contrast, Mrs J had Jacko for life. The fact that nothing had ever dented her resolve was verging on miraculous. To her, though, it needed no explanation, it was the most natural thing in the world. She needed no back-up, no injections, no rapid response teams waiting in the aisles. To paraphrase the Beatles, Mrs J knew that no matter what, all Jacko really needed, was love.

The last thing that Jacko needed, though, was a smoking ban. Over the previous months the government had initiated a ban on smoking in all forensic units, which was soon to come into play. The decision had caused uproar among many mental health care professionals, who thought it plain wrong.

As Jacko so eloquently put it: 'The geezer who dreamed up this idea is way, way crazier than me.'

The reasons the ban was flawed were obvious, according to Obi. He thought a smoking ban might spark a collective patient 'kick off'. This would then put a strain on the doctors and nurses and cause general unease in the ward. But more than anything, he thought it was wrong because smoking a cigarette is the last out and out pleasure left to a patient on a PICU.

I agreed with Obi. Mostly this ward was a vice-free world of insipid food, dreary routine and mood-stabilising meds. The one bit of autonomy – of 'I am what I am and sod the rest of you' freedom – a patient has is the right to go to the smoking room, an airless hovel near the laundry, and fire up a rolly.

Almost all those diagnosed with schizophrenia are smokers, at least in my experience. They love their cigarettes – all seven of the patients on this particular PICU did anyway. And now they were being told by some obscure quango of bureaucrats that they had to stub out their ciggies for twelve hours between 8 p.m. and 8 a.m.

Sure, if any of the patients did ever kick the habit (a big if) they would receive huge health benefits. But, to me, this was a bit like telling a homeless man he should eat his five portions of fruit and veg a day. Come on, mate, put down that Big Mac and enjoy a nice broccoli floret. He couldn't give a toss; he wants to fill his belly and enjoy it. Likewise, a psychiatric patient who is bored and frustrated wants to smoke a cigarette.

Of course, it's fair to say, none of the rest of the general public can smoke in public buildings. But they can still smoke in their own homes. They can still smoke in the street, or the park, or the garden whenever they want. No one is telling them, that for twelve hours of every day, it's illegal.

To counteract what would evidently cause a minor mutiny, the patients were all met by Alice, a petite, strawberry-blond anti-smoking adviser. Alice appeared out of her depth, but doggedly put her point across with the inevitable PowerPoint presentation. At the end of the session she produced a small nicotine cartridge and inserted it in a cigarette holder.

'This is your new cigarette,' she said proudly. She then pretended to take a long drag on it, and explained that each cartridge was the equivalent of one and a half normal cigarettes.

'You see,' she said, beaming. 'Magic!' She dragged again. 'So there it is, a smoke-free cigarette. That's what I call pure magic.'

'That's what I call a fake fag, sweetheart,' said Jacko, scowling. 'And what's the point of smoking something that has more nicotine than a cigarette? he added, not unreasonably.

He was eyeing up Alice's new smokeless cartridge with a mixture of apprehension and disgust.

'The cartridge lasts much longer,' replied Alice cheerily. 'They've proved much more effective than nicotine gum or patches in helping people stop. I think you'll be impressed.'

'I'd be more impressed by a Marlboro, sweetheart,' said Jacko, flashing a smile. 'But I'll give them a go just for you.'

The day of Alice's visit was my last on the ward. I never did find out if a smokers' mutiny occurred due to the imminent ban, but if anyone could prevent it, it would be the likes of Obi and Sally and the rest of the team.*

I remember clearly my final afternoon on the PICU. My timesheet had been signed off, I had said my farewells to the patients and staff, including a palm-stinging high five with Jacko, and was about to hand in my keys.

Just at that moment a delivery man buzzed the door. I looked at the entrance video screen and could see a burly man in a blue uniform. I left the nurses' station, greeted him and together we walked outside the unit to his van. In the boot were several boxes containing the possessions of a new patient.

On our return I buzzed open the ward door and took through one of the boxes. I dropped it off inside and was puzzled that the delivery man had not followed me with another box. When I went back outside he was sitting on one of the remaining boxes, texting.

'Aren't you going to give me a hand?' I asked. 'These boxes are pretty heavy.'

'I'm not going in there, mate!' he said, gesturing to the ward with his head. 'It's full of bloody nutters.'

'But no one's going to hurt you,' I said. 'We've got a very professional team, alarms, the lot. And if that nurse there,' I

---

*A recent survey by the Mental Health Foundation found that over 80 per cent of the respondents thought the smoking ban on psychiatric wards had not been implemented successfully. There are, as yet, no plans to reverse it.

pointed at Sally through the glass in the door, 'is able to spend five days a week here, then I'm sure you'll be OK for a couple of minutes.'

'No way, mate,' he said, handing me a box. 'I've read about people like that in the papers.'

'Oh, Sally's not that scary,' I said.

The man looked up, unsmiling. 'I ain't going anywhere near them sickos. No one's gonna make me either.'

I took the box from him, lost for words. This hulk of a man with his wrestler's torso and dagger tattoos, afraid to spend even a couple of minutes in one of the most secure units imaginable.

I was riled by his timidity and his prejudice, but mostly by the fact he didn't trust my insistence that he would be safe. I took umbrage that he didn't have faith in the ward nurses, even if he had little knowledge of their experience. And yet, I suppose he had every right to refuse — the great wuss. I didn't say anything, just nodded my head in despair.

'Tut tut all you like,' said the man, pointing at me. 'But you choose to work in there, I fucking don't.'

'Don't knock it till you've tried it,' I said, heading back into the ward with a box. 'You might be surprised.'

During our first mental health lecture The Doctor had said that part of our job as student mental health nurses was to wipe out stigma. I'd tried whenever I could but sometimes, I decided, I was just wasting my time.

That evening I joined up with Vicky, Jana and Coco for an end-of-placement drink near our nursing school.

The pub where we met was a favourite of ours, a dowdy den with a jukebox that played retro music. It was run by an ale-flushed Irishman called Seamus, who constantly gave us free drinks ('I love nurses in uniform,' he would tell us, 'even the men!'). The pub also had a couple of dogs, a lugubrious spaniel called Spam and Sausage, a half-bald dachshund.

When I turned up, the girls had already been drinking a while. They were discussing possible dissertation topics. Jana was thinking of covering the way nurses are portrayed in the media.

She was ranting – Jana gave good rant – about a recent story in which a conservative peer, Lord Mancroft, had branded nurses as 'grubby, drunken, and promiscuous'.

'What the hell does he know?' said Coco. 'He's just some stupid aristo who lives in another world.'

'To be fair, he's an ex-heroin addict,' I said. 'He's lived a bit, must have spent a bit of time within the NHS. Sure, he sounds a bit of a prat, but he's got a point. Some nurses aren't great . . . '

'He's just some silver-spooned dickhead,' interrupted Jana, banging down her pint, 'who likes to surround himself with flunkies. I mean, listen to how pompous he sounds . . . ' Jana picked up the article and began to read Lord Mancroft's comments:

'They – the nurses – talk across you as if you're not there,' she read out in her best hoity-toity accent. 'I know exactly what they got up to the night before, and how much they drank and I know exactly what they were planning to do the next night, and I can tell you, it's pretty horrifying . . . '

'Oh my god, Jimmy,' said Vicky, grabbing my arm. 'He's talking about military fitness, isn't he? You've been rumbled. It was you who cared for him.'

'No, it can't have been Jimmy,' said Jana, flicking up her beer mat. 'Lord Mancroft mentions nurses chatting to one another about their love life.' She nodded. 'Jimmy doesn't have a love life.'

'I'll have you know, ladies, I'm hoping to find my soulmate this very night.'

'Oh, so where are you and Lord Mancroft dining then?'

'Very funny, Vicky.'

'Can we please get back to my dissertation,' said Jana. 'Do you think the media would make a good subject?'

'It's a brilliant one,' I said, picking up her newspaper. 'You can talk about Lord Mancroft slagging off nurses, putting them under one umbrella. And how about that Christian nurse who was told she couldn't say a prayer to a sick patient? She'd be good.'

'Or that poor nurse who made a video at that grim nursing home and got struck off for her efforts,' said Coco. 'She should have been given a medal, not lost her job.'

'Yes, it's a good subject isn't it?' said Jana, already imagining her academic plaudits. 'I really need something to cheer me up, you know. I've been getting so pissed off with the course recently.'

'Second-year blues,' I said. 'All our group are going through it, too. Fed up with writing essays, fed up with repetitive lectures. We just want to qualify. The end seems so far off.'

'Too right,' said Jana. 'And my current placement is horrible. My mentor is a complete cow. She does nothing, sits gossiping in the nurses' station and gets me to do everything.'

'Yeah, my mentor is a bitch, too,' sympathised Coco. 'She's just so jaded. I have no idea why she's still in nursing. She seems to hate the patients.'

'Maybe Lord Mancroft had a point,' I said. 'I've worked with mostly wonderful nurses, but let's face it, there's some rotten ones, too.'

'We all know there's a few rotten nurses,' said Vicky. 'But most of us are fine. We don't need some stuck-up ex-junkie to tell us we're all useless. The job is hard enough as it is.'

'I propose a toast,' said Jana, raising her glass, and lighting up with a smile. 'Up yours, Lord Mancroft!'

At this stage Seamus, his cheeks glowing red, appeared with a round of drinks. He looked like a benevolent Falstaff, the drinks tray balancing on his magnificent paunch. 'These are all on me,' he announced. 'To nurses, God bless you all.' How Seamus made any money I don't know, he seemed to spend all his time buying his punters rounds.

'To nurses,' said Vicky, raising her glass. 'And lovely land-lords.' We charged our glasses, drank and then cheered, which set Spam and Sausage off barking. Jana stroked Spam, whose tail began to wag furiously. She picked him up and balanced him on her knee.

'At least someone appreciates me,' said Jana, kissing the top of Spam's head. 'Sometimes I think nursing is the toughest job in the world, you know. And the pay is dire. I'm really tempted to quit sometimes.'

'Come on, Jana,' said Vicky. 'You're a great nurse. You're just having a bad placement. You'll feel better about the next one.'

I had to leave at this stage, but was worried about how down Jana sounded. Despite her natural cynicism she was a devoted and very capable student, who usually weathered any rough patches. But that night she wasn't herself at all.

Buoyed by my drink at Seamus's tavern I pedalled off to a birth-day knees-up for Maggie, the Amazonian trainee teacher I'd fallen for during my nursery placement. Since she had written her number in my leaving card weeks ago, she had been too busy to meet up. Now, finally, I could see her.

The party venue was even more of a dive than Seamus's joint. When I parked my bike outside, Maggie rushed over, grabbed it and brought it into the bar area. 'It will get nicked in no time out there,' she insisted. 'It's safer here. The barman won't mind, he's a friend.'

Things were in full swing. Some of the girls were singing a spirited version of 'Hit Me Baby One More Time'. Vodka shots were being slugged. I joined a group table with Maggie and several others. Fred, the head teacher, shook my hand and told me he was just leaving.

'Good to see you again, Jimmy,' Fred said, heading for the door. 'I'm sorry, I'm too old for all this . . . ' He gestured at the ambient mayhem. 'More of a Sinatra man.'

Maggie and I were shouting to make our voices heard above the Britney wanabes. Maggie was telling me how much she was enjoying her teacher training, but was finding the paperwork overwhelming.

'Did you know, Jimmy,' she bellowed in my ear, 'four out of ten trainee teachers drop out before they even make it to the classroom. It's so hard at times.' Clearly nurses weren't the only ones with the tough agenda.

'Sometimes I really need to let off steam,' yelled Maggie. 'Come on, let's dance.'

We joined the throng of other teachers on the small, jam-packed dance floor. Hits by Queen and Oasis were blasting out. Maggie, in her high heels, was a half foot taller than me but we jived around happily together. I was punching way above my weight (and height) with her: she was gorgeous. We certainly made an incongruous pair. She tall, black and lavishly dread-locked, I stocky, white with a short back and sides.

After several more dances the music dried up and the barman called last orders. Everyone sang 'Happy Birthday' to Maggie one more time before we filtered out on the streets. I waited while she hugged her friends and colleagues goodbye. When it was just me and her, I told her I would be honoured to walk her home. There was a pause. Making any sort of romantic move in your thirties is always toe-curlingly awkward, and ripe for humiliation, even after a Jack Daniels or two. I braced myself for the polite but inevitable brush-off.

'Sure you can walk me home,' said Maggie, grabbing my arm. 'I live just round the block.' Oh my God! This was like a gift from heaven. One minute I had been ridiculed for my sad-sack singledom and now here I was, strutting out with my Amazonian princess into the starry night. OK, there weren't any stars, just a jaundiced wedge of moon, but, hey, I didn't care; with Maggie on my arm anywhere felt like the Champs Elysées.

Maggie really did live just round the corner and we made it in less than five minutes. I locked my bike in the communal stairwell of her tower block.

'Follow me,' said Maggie. She sashayed gracefully up two flights of stairs to her apartment and pushed open the door. I followed her into the sitting room, full of jungly palms and a faint smell of Maggie's perfume. A large map of the Caribbean was splayed across the wall. Maggie leant against the sofa.

'So, it's been a great evening, Maggie, thanks for . . . '

She put a finger over my lips. 'You gonna get on tiptoes and kiss me, Jimmy?'

My heart bashed against my rib cage in a visceral high five. 'Can you kick off your heels first?' I suggested.

'You'd still need to tiptoe even then, big man.'

I arched my Doc Martens to their maximum reach and sank into her beautiful face. I was overcome by her smell, an intoxicating blend of musk and earth and sweetness. I was high on it, as if I hadn't smelt anything properly for years. Her cantilevered cleavage was now squeezed tight into my chest: it felt as if she had about ten heartbeats. We continued to totter around the room in a comic last-dance-at-the-disco routine, before tumbling on to the sofa. Maggie began to undo my shirt, while I kissed her neck, my hands running through her dreadlocks, savouring their softness, their unfamiliarity.

'Mum!' A voice came from the other side of the sofa. I sprung up, shirt akimbo, and saw a boy of about five looking up at me.

'Who are you?' said the boy. 'Who are you!' I thought. I looked at him, looked at Maggie and then back at the boy.

Maggie manoeuvred herself from under me and rolled off the sofa.

'This is Jimmy, Sam,' she said, straightening out her hair. 'Don't worry, he's a friend of mine.'

'Hi, Sam,' I said, frantically putting my shirt back on. He continued to stare at me, unashamedly, in the way only a five-year-old can. A few seconds later he was joined by another boy, almost identical, except a year or so younger.

'Joseph!' said Maggie. 'What are you doing up?'

'Who's he, mum?' said Joseph, pointing at me.

'That's Jimmy.'

'Hi, Joseph,' I said. I gave him a quick wave as I continued to wrestle with my shirt. Both Sam and Joseph continued to stare at me, this half-dressed stranger on their sofa.

Another Caribbean woman burst through the door. She was about Maggie's age and looked very distraught.

'Argghh,' she screamed as she saw me. Was my chest hair really that bad?

'Clara, this is Jimmy, a friend of mine.'

'Hi, Clara.'

Clara looked me up and down (mostly down), and grinned at Maggie.

'So sorry, Maggs,' Clara said. 'I wouldn't have let the boys disturb you if I'd known you had company. They couldn't sleep.'

'No worries, babe,' said Maggie. 'How's little Charise?'

'Oh, she's cool. Sleeping away.'

I was slowly doing some arithmetic. Sam, Joseph and little Charise. Maggie was a mother of three. The only person left out of this mix was the father. He was bound to be the next to enter, stage left, probably with a meat cleaver.

Maggie and Clara ushered the boys back into their bedroom. I prepared to make a hasty exit, but just as I was heading for the door Maggie reappeared.

'Sorry, Jimmy, I shouldn't have put you through that,' she said, kissing me. 'There's no father by the way, he's no longer with us. I wasn't messing you around. And Clara's just a dear friend who babysat for the evening. I hardly ever get out, you see. This was a big night for me.'

'It's OK, Maggie, really. I understand. But, hey, in the light of everything, I probably better head off.'

'Why not sleep on the sofa and leave in the morning? You don't want to pedal back right now, do you?'

I thought about her offer for about one and a half seconds. 'OK, sure, good idea.'

Maggie vanished to tend her children. I fell asleep on the sofa and woke up shortly before dawn. Maggie was sleeping by my side. She was still in last night's clothes, one arm on my chest. She looked beautiful.

I kissed her face and stood up. 'You leaving me, big man?' she asked, opening an eye.

'I better go before the kids wake up.'

'Yeah, OK.' She grabbed my leg and pulled me towards her. 'You're not my usual type, Jimmy, but thank you for a lovely night.' She smiled. 'I won't see you again, big man. You ain't ready to cope with three kids, and you and me are different as hell. Me all direct and street-smart and you all English and polite. But we had a fun time, hey, Jimmy?'

'One of the best,' I said. 'It's a night I'll never forget.' The French have a great expression, *l'esprit d'escalier*, meaning the thing you wished you'd said when descending the staircase, the missed riposte, the forgotten *bon mot*, the goodbye left hanging. As usual I couldn't rustle up anything remotely poignant, so I simply kissed Maggie and told her she was 'really great'. Lord Byron would have turned in his grave. Even Lord Mancroft might have been more eloquent.

Maggie flashed me one of her heart-thumping smiles and glided off to check on her children. She was right, I never would see her again, but I would often think of her.

I pedalled back to my flat like a man possessed. It was springtime and birdsong and blossom were in the air. I felt like a teenager, singing, punching the air with delight. This nursing course was hard for sure, but it had moments of splendour, and

Maggie's warm fingertips on my face had felt like balm, like some strange reward.

Sometimes it's only when you've been touched in the right way that you realise how lonely you've been.

Chapter 12

CLAY RAINBOWS

I turned up at my next placement still with a spring in my step after my tryst with Maggie. Monday morning always felt better if you'd been lying in someone's arms over the weekend, even if it was on a clapped-out sofa, with regular interruptions from two toddlers and a hysterical babysitter. But this was no time for revelling in Maggie's afterglow, I was about to be brought crashing back down to earth.

'You must be the student,' said BB, my new mentor, as I stood at her office door. She was a lanky, middle-aged woman, who looked as if she'd applied her lipstick on a trampoline. 'Ever done a depot injection, new boy?'

'Er, no, not yet'.

'Hell's bells, you should have injected someone by now.' BB eyed me over her horn-rimmed glasses. 'You're near the end of your second year. You need to inject!'

'Well, I'm happy to have a stab at it.'

'Oh, God, we've got a joker on our hands,' said BB, rolling her eyes. 'Next you'll be needling me, or telling me to look sharp. Trust me, I've heard every injection pun in the book, you little prick.' Actually, she didn't say those last three words, but the tone of her voice strongly implied them.

'Anyway, Timmy, Jimmy whatever your name is,' added BB. 'You can join Dougal this afternoon, he's the injection king.'

Before the afternoon's jabs with Dougal, BB gave me a tour of the office. It felt strange to be at a placement that wasn't a ward. This building, with its neat desks and filing cabinets, looked more like a firm of accountants than a mental health facility. I mentioned this to BB.

'Yes, you have a point,' she stated, coolly. 'But not many accountants wear jeans, have access to controlled drugs, or their receptionist shielded by reinforced glass.' She glowered at me. 'With the possible exception of Enron's.'

BB explained the role of our nursing team was to visit the most mentally vulnerable people in the community. They had a mixture of illnesses – schizophrenia, depression, personality disorder, alcohol or drug addiction. Many needed to be seen daily, others only once a fortnight.

In the medication room BB showed me cupboards full of drugs – antidepressants, antipsychotics and the odd packet of vitamins. She plucked out a depot injection pack from the fridge for me to look at. Depots were used as a substitute for pills, releasing medication slowly into the bloodstream.

'Feast your eyes on that, new boy,' BB ordered, flicking the syringe. The needle on it looked long enough to knit with. Having been quite gung-ho about the prospect of injecting, I was now gripped by fear. With a needle that size I'd have to be as deadeyed as William Tell.

'Depot injections are intramuscular and you stick them here,' said BB, prodding at her expansive bottom.

'Oh, don't get all shy on me,' said BB, as I retreated. 'I'll draw you a diagram.' She ripped a sheet of paper from a notepad and began to doodle a picture of a human backside.

'You have to stick the needle right there!' BB stabbed the diagram to the side of the sketched buttock. 'In the upper outer quadrant.

'If you screw up and hit here, near the centre,' BB jabbed at the drawing again, 'or here, near to the cleft you might hit the sciatic nerve! That runs up to the brain. Do that and you might even paralyse someone.' She scowled at me. 'In fact, do that, and I'll paralyse you!' She and Mr Temple should get together. I'm sure there must be a dating site: mentorfromhell.com

'Don't worry,' I reassured her. 'I won't paralyse any patients.'

'Any what?'

'Patients,' I said more slowly.

'And who are patients?'

This was getting silly. 'Patients are the people we care for.'

'They're not patients!' shouted BB, her cheeks reddening. 'They are clients! Don't you read the papers. We call them clients now.' This place was becoming more like an accountant's office every minute.

'But calling them clients makes them sound like people we do business with, not care for,' I said, standing my ground. 'Patient sounds much better.'

'It's client, OK! Client makes them feel more empowered. If I hear you say patient again I shan't be happy.'

I tried to imagine BB ever being happy, but soon gave up. What did BB stand for anyway? Ball Breaker? Or was it an ironic take on Bambi? She certainly possessed the horns, if not antlers.

'That's the end of the tour,' BB told me, turning on her heel. 'The last student dropped out after only a week. Let's hope you do better. Now go and find Dougal.'

Dougal couldn't have been more different from BB. He was a genial man with a stooped posture and swept-back silvery blond hair. On his back was a large green knapsack full of medication, which made him resemble a world-weary tortoise. He clearly was, as BB said, the 'injection king'.

'Oh, so you're joining me this afternoon,' Dougal said, in his daydreamy Scottish accent. 'What fun! It will be nice to have the company.' He made it sound as if we were off to have a picnic in the park.

'Have you injected anyone before?' he asked, taking a file from the landslide of papers on his desk.

'Only cows and sheep on some farms I've worked on,' I said. 'Never a human being.'

'Oh, very good, I'm sure that will help.' He looked into the middle distance as if in a reverie. 'I think I'd rather enjoy injecting a cow.'

'Dougal loves injecting,' said Gina, a young, bespectacled social worker at the desk opposite. 'If a client doesn't want their jab, Dougal can always persuade them.'

That afternoon Dougal, Gina and I were due to visit three clients. All of them suffered from schizophrenia and needed a depot injection to combat their psychosis.

We caught a succession of buses – the office had no cars – to the home of our first client, a Somali man called Hanzi, who wasn't in. It was just as well we turned up, though. Dougal pushed open the door to Hanzi's bedsit to be greeted by a cloud of smoke. A saucepan on the stove had been left on full heat and an acrid smell of burnt chemicals filled the air. Whatever had been cooking had dried up ages ago and turned to soot. Gina turned off the gas and covered her nose.

The flat was a war zone with beer cans and cigarette packets everywhere. There were also lots of khat leaves – a mild stimulant, chewed by many Somalis – carpeting the floor. Although khat is illegal in several European countries, the UK had yet to ban it.

'We haven't seen Hanzi for almost a week,' said Gina, waving her hands around to disperse the smoke. 'That's bad news. His behaviour's pretty wild, slamming doors, yelling at nurses. He really needs his jab. If he carries on like this he'll be sectioned.'

Dougal explained that clients were often not at home. The team wasted lots of time this way, but, as many of the clients didn't have telephones, visiting was the only way to check up on them.

'Visiting means we cover our arses if anything goes wrong,' said Gina. 'If we make an effort, no one can say we aren't doing our jobs.'

We had better luck with the next client, Amar, a Sikh, who lived in his parents' large, chi-chi apartment half a mile from Hanzi. Amar had a stubbly, angular face, incongruous with his fleshy physique. He said very little, and seemed to agree with whatever his father, a sharp-tongued retired soldier in a blue turban, told him. Despite being over thirty, Amar came across like a teenager.

Dougal told me he would carry out Amar's injection himself, but that I could do the next.

'You watch and learn, Jimmy,' said Gina, smiling. She had a kind, reassuring smile, and floral tattoos that straddled her sandalled feet. She could pass as a folk singer circa 1972. Like many social workers in the team, she had a very casual dress sense.

We looked on as Dougal unpacked the syringe, the needle, a Band-Aid and some latex gloves. He worked with the slow precision of a bomb defuser.

On request Amar pulled down his trousers, Dougal plunged the needle into his client's ample backside, injected the Haliperidol, pulled out the syringe and put on the plaster. It all took about five seconds, and looked a cinch.

'Didn't feel a thing,' said Amar, happily.

'See, Jimmy,' said Dougal, as we left. 'Piece of cake.'

Our final call of the day was a short walk from Amar's place. We arrived just as the sun was dropping over a row of cherry trees across the street, resplendent in their late-spring bloom.

Gina knocked on our client's door. When no one answered she began to bellow: 'Come on, John. I can hear you in there.' Soon after, a fortyish man with a haunted look ushered us in.

John lived in a grim, damp-walled lair that was so full of junk, so rotten and forlorn, that it seemed to sag before our eyes.

There were photos everywhere. I noticed one of John on a shelf, kissing a pretty, moon-faced woman in a wedding dress. They both looked about twenty years old. Another showed John as a young man, leaning against a car, tanned and happy.

It was hard to recognise the John of today from these photos. His once bushy hairline had receded dramatically, his face now pallid and drooped. The saddest of his photos were of his young daughter, a tomboy with sapphire eyes: as a baby, at school, going off to a party in a spangly dress. She was all over the room. But, according to Dougal, John hadn't seen her for years, or his ex-wife or anyone really – just psychiatric nurses wielding needles.

'Hi, John, this is Jimmy,' said Dougal. 'Do you mind if he does your injection this afternoon?'

'Why are there three of you?' John asked, confused. For reasons of safety the team always did community visits in twos: three was more unusual.

'Because Jimmy's a student,' said Gina. 'He's got to learn to inject. You'd be doing him a real favour.'

'Oh, OK then.' John looked at me. 'Just make sure you don't mess it up.'

'Don't worry.' I was tempted to tell him I'd had experience injecting cows but decided against it.

I started to unpack the Haliperidol syringe. With all eyes on me, I was mortified to find my hands were shaking. Thankfully, John turned his back at this point. He began fiddling with his belt, ready to lower his trousers.

'Calm down, Jimmy,' Gina whispered, seeing my shaking hands. She put a hand on my arm.

I took a few deep breaths but continued to resemble a malaria victim. I couldn't believe how much my hands were shaking. God, this was embarrassing. I was so glad John couldn't see me. After several aborted attempts to screw the syringe and the needle together, I finally succeeded. I then shook it up and held it like a dart, ready to plunge it into John's upper outer quadrant.

Back at college we'd only had one brief lesson on how to do injections. It involved jabbing syringes into a dummy that supposedly had 'authentically human skin'. In fact its skin was less human, and more rhino. I'd struggled so much to inject the needle, I'd needed to use both hands. Mr Temple, with characteristic menace, told us we had it lucky. 'When I trained to inject we had to practise on oranges! Oranges! You lot have got it soft.'

Now, here I was, about to inject my first real client. I'm not usually squeamish but for some reason was overwhelmed by nerves. The fact the needle appeared a finger-length long – we're talking ET's finger here – was scary. The fact John's cheek was small and skinny didn't help either, unlike Amar's meatier target.

I knelt on the floor, took aim, said a quick prayer (please God, let me miss the sciatic nerve) and plunged the needle deep into John's buttock. He flinched. I pushed in the liquid Haliperidol, checked I hadn't hit a vein and then pulled away the needle. A little gush of blood streamed out. In a panic I used several alcoholic wipes to clean it up, before putting on a Band Aid, and throwing the needle in a sharp's box. I was still shaking as I went to wash my hands.

'Thanks for letting me do that, John,' I said, as I came out of the washroom.

'That's all right,' replied John. 'But do I really have to keep having these bloody injections?'

'It's either that or tablets,' chipped in Dougal, who explained to John that in the past he had forgotten his tablets and that the injection was slow release, lasted two weeks, and meant he didn't have to worry about pills.

'But I can't get horny now,' said John, gesturing south with his eyes. 'I'm as limp as a lettuce leaf down there. Flaccido bloody Domingo.'

Many antipsychotic drugs had side effects, including a loss of libido. Dougal later told me John complained about his waning libido every time he was seen. Tragically, he was still hoping his wife would return, even though they split up more than a decade earlier, and she had not seen him since.

Once we were out of the door I let out a long sigh.

'Don't worry, Jimmy,' Dougal stressed. 'I shook during my first injection, too. You did OK. At least you didn't kill him, hey.'

Even though Dougal was joking, I was still anxious I might have hurt John. I really had been shaking uncontrollably. Frankly, I was ashamed of myself.

When we got back to the office, I wrote up my notes and furtively made a phone call to John. He was one of the few clients with a mobile phone, at least one of the few prepared to answer it. It sounds ridiculous now, but I wanted to make sure he was still alive.

'Hello . . . hello. Who's this?' John sounded deeply suspicious.

'Oh hello, John,' I said. 'This is Jimmy, the student nurse, just confirming the team are due to see you in a couple of weeks.'

'I know they are. They always do. I'm not stupid, you know.'

'And are you feeling OK, John?'

'No, like a piece of shit.' *Oh no, I'd hit his sciatic nerve!* 'But a bit better than yesterday.' *Phew, thank you God.*

'Very good, John. Bye now.'

How ridiculous to have phoned John. Of course he was all right, I was acting like a jerk. But I was relieved to learn when I spoke to Kiko – a man who had been in the Senegalese army, no less – that he had shaken during his first depot injection, too. He'd even followed his client around the ward for a couple of hours afterwards to check he didn't peg out.

As Dougal told me, a depot injection was a rite of passage. I'd got through it, just about, and when I performed my next injection was thankfully blessed with hands as steady as a neuro-surgeon's.

The following morning I did another visit with Gina. It was pouring with rain, the sky the colour of faded denim. We weaved through town, huddled together under Gina's umbrella, engrossed in discussing the differences between a social worker and a nurse.

'You guys deal more with the drugs,' said Gina, jumping a puddle. 'We deal with welfare, housing, benefits, that kind of stuff.'

'But you are dropping off pills today.'

'The roles do blend at times,' she explained. 'If I'm snowed under I might get a nurse to help me with paperwork, too.'

We ducked under a bus shelter, the rain so heavy everyone had begun to seek cover. I asked Gina if she enjoyed her job.

'You know, Jimmy, since that Baby P case, hardly anyone wants to be a social worker. Did you see all the headlines at the time?' Gina paused and shook her umbrella dry. 'Mistakes were made, sure, really bad ones. Poor kid. But it was such a witch-hunt. Doctors, nurses, and therapists saw Baby P, too. They got off lightly. It was social workers who really took the rap for his death – splashed over the tabloids like criminals.'

Gina shook her head. 'It's not surprising there's a massive shortage of us now. If we stamp down too hard, we get called fascists, and if we go in too soft, we're called cop-outs. We can't win.' She shrugged her shoulders. 'We get paid shit money, for shitloads of responsibility. But hey, someone's got to do it.'

'Have you thought of leaving?' I asked.

She started to laugh. 'Hey, sorry, Jimmy. You're all new and dewy eyed, I shouldn't try to change that. I do like my job really, it just eats me up sometimes.' She tapped her forehead. 'Mental health work can do that. You'll find out soon enough.'

A half hour later we arrived at a day centre for homeless people. One of Gina's clients, Leanne, was a regular, and she wanted to check up on her. Leanne had been homeless for years, and although Gina had tried to get her into accommodation in the past, she'd kept going back to the street.

'Leanne's bipolar,' explained Gina. 'Zooms between the

North Pole, happy as hell, and the South Pole, desperately sad. She never knows how long she'll be at either place. She's sometimes in denial she's ill at all.'

'Sounds tricky,' I said.

Gina rolled her eyes at me. 'Leanne's a character, lovely and all, but she can be a right pain in the butt.'

I mooched about at reception while Gina had an initial meeting with Leanne. I noticed that most of the guests wandering around the homeless centre were male. I'd read somewhere that male rough-sleepers outnumber females ten to one.

Just as I was about to start my second coffee, Gina called me. She introduced Leanne, and went off to make a phone call, leaving her client and me to continue chin-wagging.

Leanne was gaunt, with skin the colour of wet sugar, but she still retained a glimmer of her former beauty – she'd once been a model – that which hadn't been drained away by depression, alcohol and domestic abuse.

'Did you know, darling,' said Leanne, blowing on a hot chocolate, her eyes suspended in nets of red wire, 'that my husband ruined me?'

Leanne explained that her husband used to beat her all the time, and stopped her from modelling because it made him jealous. Leanne put up with the violence for several years, before deciding to escape. She bolted one weekend and moved in with a girlfriend. Despite initial euphoria, Leanne soon slipped into depression and an increasing reliance on gin. Her friend couldn't handle her. She moved out, holing up in a hostel and, finally, the street.

'It all happened so quickly, darling,' she said. 'One minute I was a model.' She tossed back her lank, mousy hair. 'I did shoots for cosmetics, not catwalk stuff. But still, it was good money. I had lots of friends. Next thing I'm in the marriage from hell, then – ka boom! On the street! Alone! It was all so depressing.' She swigged on an imaginary bottle. 'It can happen to anyone, darling, even classy girls like me. You chase your rainbow but don't find gold at the end of it, just clay! Clay rainbows, darling, the story of my life.'

'Not clay rainbows again, Leanne.' Gina reappeared. 'You crazy woman!' This comment tickled Leanne and she laughed, a high-pitched and contagious sound. I noticed Gina had a much more informal relationship with her clients than many of the nurses.

Before we left Gina booked Leanne into a nearby night shelter, and told her one of the team's nurses would visit that evening. We said our goodbyes and walked out into the street. The rain had stopped but there were puddles everywhere.

'Leanne's calm at the moment,' said Gina, as we made our way back to the office. 'But when she's manic she gets deluded and thinks she's Kate Moss.' Gina pouted her lips for emphasis. 'One week she was even convinced she was Lady Diana. Of course, she's ecstatic when she's manic. But then come the lows, and they are really bad.'

Gina explained the depression had struck Leanne in her prime, her early twenties. Her husband had probably turned violent because he couldn't cope. She did well to escape him. Domestic violence happens to one in four women and leads to a lot of homelessness.

'Don't people like Leanne sometimes enjoy their mania?' I asked. 'Refuse their medication because the highs are so great?'

'The highs can be towering,' admitted Gina, exhaling a plume of smoke. 'But tend to be short-lived. And the crashes in mood are devastating. The meds can work wonders but it's not an illness I'd wish on anyone.' She smiled sadly. 'That's why Leanne talks about clay rainbows. It's a brilliant description of bipolar, actually.' Gina arched her hands in the shape of a rainbow. 'All that glorious hope, colour and promise and then – phut!' She flicked away her cigarette. 'It can suddenly turn to clay.'

I enjoyed my visits with Gina, hearing things from a social worker's perspective, but most of my time was spent charging after BB. Everyone charged after BB. She power-walked her way between visits, shunning all forms of public transport, and expected everyone to keep up. For all her frostiness towards students, I was glad to see she was much sunnier with her patients – 'It's clients, new boy, clients!'

BB's home life sounded challenging to say the least. She had a long-term female partner, and between them they had three children, two adopted boys from China, and BB's own daughter, who had been fathered by a gay friend of hers. Her life made *EastEnders* sound like *The Last of the Summer Wine*. BB's mobile would trill constantly throughout the day, calls from the office or home, asking for her advice, her presence, her time. Her capacity to juggle was verging on heroic. Despite the fact she breathed fire and always called me 'new boy', I had started to warm to her. She was certainly a good, if unconventional, nurse.

I remember one morning we visited a client of BB's called Raj. BB had filled me in on him before the visit.

Raj was originally from India, a chubby man in his early sixties, who suffered from paranoid schizophrenia. He spent much of his time walking the streets. BB was a great advocate of walking. She believed it was Raj's pounding of pavements, more than his medication, that kept his demons at bay.

Raj was a genuine lone wolf. He never spoke of his early life in India, and seemed to have no links to anyone or anything. His one friend had been an old lady, who had died a year ago. Raj had been bereft ever since. Using a photo of the old lady's face, some of her clothes and a pair of her shoes, he had created a shrine for her on the floor of his hostel room.

BB was the only person Raj was prepared to open up to, and even then, only slightly. I noticed she softened her normal machine-gun voice to fit in with Raj's coy drawl. His English was very limited, so much so that he spoke only in the present tense. This was oddly fitting, as Raj never mentioned his past or future anyway.

Raj's current problem was his personal hygiene. Other than when he took the odd shower, he had not removed his shirt for weeks. The already threadbare garment had begun not only to smell, but to fray.

The head nurse at the hostel was concerned. Raj's behaviour in every other aspect had been fine, but his shirt was becoming a fixation. He believed if he didn't wear it, people would die, and nothing would shake him free from this notion. BB had been called in as a last resort.

After a brief discussion with Raj, BB told me to dash off and buy a couple of cheap shirts, as similar as possible to Raj's current one, to try to tempt him to change it. Within twenty minutes I came back with a pair of Primark specials, but Raj point blank refused to wear them. BB, to my horror, then recommended my shirt, a sort of purply lumberjack job.

'That shirt good!' said Raj, pointing at me.

BB took me to one side. 'Well done, new boy,' she stated. 'Raj obviously admires your gay cowboy look.'

'Gay cowboy – this shirt's from Millets . . .'

'Shut up and listen. Just nip to the washroom, rip off your shirt and swap it with one of the new ones you bought. The staff here can wash your purple one later and give it to Raj.'

'But I like this shirt!'

'Do it, new boy, or I'll have to give him mine.' I looked at BB's top, a fusion of Laura Ashley and lace with lapels so wide they could take flight.

'Your top is a bit too cutting edge, BB,' I said.

'Shut it, new boy, he clearly wants your shirt – it's his own he thinks will kill people.' She took hold of my collar. 'Personally speaking, wearing this, this . . . sartorial horror, would kill me – with sheer embarrassment. But he likes it. So rip it off. Now!'

BB's hunch was right and on our next visit to see Raj he was happily sporting my old shirt – no longer afraid his dress sense would hurt anyone.

A few days later I found a new check shirt on my desk, courtesy of BB. On it was a note. 'Thanks, new boy, Raj is important to me and you helped him. Hope you like this new shirt. I decided the Brokeback Mountain look suits you.'

What was good about working with BB was that she never treated the clients like victims. As with Gina, she was straight-talking and professional, but unafraid to share a joke with them or poke some fun. I noticed BB had a strong rapport with all her long-term clients, especially a larger than life lady called Joanna.

I met Joanna on several occasions over the following weeks. Along with bouts of depression she was thought to have a histrionic personality disorder, an illness caused by a crushing lack of self-worth. At times this was hard to believe, as Joanna was a bubbly, blue-eyed blonde; a loud, chaotic, and often joyous force of nature.

Granted, Joanna was no picnic. She had a long history of drink and drug abuse. She constantly needed approval, craved excitement and regularly flashed her body at strangers. She could be manipulative and inappropriate, often wearing the skimpiest of outfits. She was hugely overweight, and needed regular insulin jabs for her diabetes.

'For all her faults,' BB once told me. 'I think Joanna is magnificent.'

And she was, too. The first time I met Joanna was when BB, Gina and I took her out to a coffee shop. Within ten minutes Joanna had flashed a breast at me, and asked me to marry her. Later she took off her blond wig to reveal her pallid, balding pate. Gina and BB told her to stop, which she did, but they were also unable to control their smiles. Joanna constantly pushed boundaries, but there was something so natural, so untamed about her, you could not help but be won over.

Mental health nursing is often a hugely earnest profession, so it is important to take the laughs when you get them. And, for all the sadness of Joanna's illness, there were moments of joy, too.

One morning BB, Dougal and I were due to visit Joanna's hostel with some fresh medication. We'd already heard from the staff there that Joanna had been banned from going out. She had apparently spent all her benefit money on drink, then come back late at night, semi-naked and roaring drunk, leading her to smash her bedroom mirror. She'd then fallen into a deep sleep.

By the time we arrived Joanna had woken and was raising hell, shouting and flailing her arms around. BB was forced to take her to one side. Together they sat on the hostel's stairs and talked things through, while Dougal and I stood watching at the hostel door.

'I want a man,' I could hear Joanna saying. 'Or just a hug, BB. You know what I mean. Why can't I have nobody?' I could hear BB trying to placate her.

Then, out of nowhere Joanna charged at Dougal and me. 'I want a hug!' she declared. It seemed either Dougal or I would do. She clearly wasn't fussy. The situation was straight out of the Marx brothers, Joanna squashing Dougal and me against the front door, with BB dementedly trying to pull her away.

Joanna's weight enveloped me, keeping me pinned to the door while Dougal managed to slide away. BB doggedly wrestled with Joanna, hauling at her shoulders. Some of the hostel's nursing staff soon caught wind of the commotion and came rushing to help.

Joanna was not aggressive but her hug was certainly tight. Her jumper was pressed hard against me, letting off smells of rain, smoke and stale sweat. As she was being pulled away from me, Joanna kept shouting: 'I just want a hug. A hug. A hug.' Finally, exhausted by the tug of war with all of us, she collapsed back down on the stair, her head in her hands. Her blond wig was ruffled and askew. For a few seconds there was silence, and it looked as though Joanna was in tears. Then her head shot up, a huge smile lit her face, and she began to laugh: great, deep, uncontrollable laughter.

One of the hostel's nurses began trying to reprimand her. 'Joanna, this is unacceptable, this craving attention . . . ' But BB was already in fits, and it wasn't long before Dougal and I joined in. The hostel staff soon followed suit, all of us in gales of laughter.

'Man, I need a cigarette,' said Joanna, after we were all spent. 'It took time for us all to calm down. We had no doubt flouted all the mental health guidelines, laughing away like fools. But Joanna's need for a hug was so spontaneous, so human, it was hard to be too punitive. BB was instinctive and professional, and knew when to discipline and when to let things go. She'd known Joanna for a decade and sensed, in this case, that laughter was the best medicine. Joanna knew she'd misbehaved; there was little point in dragging it out.

After a debrief and a quick farewell to Joanna, we walked back to the office. On the way I reflected about Joanna's desperate need for a hug. At the time it had seemed so absurd, so comic, her running headlong at two men, enveloping us in her ample embrace. Of course, it was only right for Dougal and me to push her away, but was Joanna's behaviour so surprising?

I thought back to my recent night with Maggie, how just being held by her had felt so special. I had so many people in my life – Poppin, my parents, my siblings, my friends. Some would be happy to hug me, many less so, but they were all there for me in their different ways.

The tragedy of mental illness is that it often destroys *all* friendships and severs *all* family ties for those suffering from it. Of course, there are those people, like Jacko's mother, whose love remains unconditional. But for all the Mrs Js, there are plenty of parents, siblings, partners, and friends who just can't cope.

Like so many of the mentally ill, Joanna had nobody – except paid professionals – willing to handle her. And, looking at her situation coldly, she probably never would. No one to love her. No one to hug her. But Joanna still had the spirit to laugh, to seek affection, to squeeze whatever she could from life (including Dougal and me) despite her limited circumstances.

'You know, sometimes I'm envious of Joanna,' said BB, once we were back at the office. 'Sure, her life is sad in many ways, but she's so guileless, so unaffected. She's hell to handle but there's such a purity about her. Like she's thrown away her mask.' BB spread her arms, imitating Joanna's hug. 'What do you reckon, new boy? Can any sane person be that honest? That free?'

BB, despite her sharp (at times forked) tongue, was a formidable teacher. She stretched me, asked me things I'd never have considered myself, and let me help with her more challenging clients. I was nearing the end of the second year now, and in the third year needed to select my sign-off mentor – someone who would assess me as professionally competent, unleash me into the scary world of the fully qualified nurse.

It was possible for me to choose any of my past mentors – Tony, Obi, Sally – but I was particularly enjoying my community placement and plumped for BB, whose maverick style I had come to find refreshing.

'Oh shit, new boy,' said BB, rolling her eyes, when I told her. 'I hoped I'd scared you off. No student's asked me to be a sign-off mentor before. I suppose I better agree.' She pulled down her glasses and gave me a stare. 'Just make sure you buy me plenty of doughnuts. And flatter me constantly.'

I was excited about BB's mentorship, and about entering my final year. But, in truth, I still wondered if I had done the right thing, swapping from children's nursing to mental health.

On reflection, I had often found nursing on mental health wards frustrating. At times it seemed we were shielding patients from the outside world, not preparing them to get back in it. We gave them their medication, served them their food, and bar the odd tai chi lesson or game of pool, offered precious little stimulation. Everything was done for them.

Much of the time patients on the wards sat around watching TV and smoking. A few took advantage of the therapists, cooking classes, gym sessions and ward meetings, but many just seemed to be going to seed. Despite the best efforts of the staff, mental health wards were not always empowering environments. And I'd worked on some of the better ones. I had visited Kiko at one of his placements on a ward that had only one small window to let in the light. It looked dark and demoralising.

'This place is hell, Jimmy,' Kiko told me. 'Worst place ever for your mental health. I come home each day feeling like shit. I dread to think what it's like for the patients.'

In contrast to the wards, I enjoyed the community placement's outdoorsy element and hustle bustle. But it wasn't without its shocks, too. I'd been staggered, perhaps naively, by the huge numbers of mentally ill people mouldering away in bedsits and hostels, by the sheer levels of loneliness and despair out there.

As BB's team of nurses each had to visit up to a dozen homes a day it meant little time for individual clients. Often it was simply a quick: 'Hello. How are you? Take your medication. Fill in this form. Everything OK? See you next time,' and then off we'd rush to the next visit. Longer visits tended to take place only in emergencies. Every day we seemed to be putting a metaphorical Band Aid on all our clients, but never getting to the root of their problems.

I explained this to BB one morning at handover.

'This isn't *Grey's Anatomy*, new boy,' she said. 'What did you expect? Nurse Jimmy wiping out mental illness in a few months?' She wagged a finger at me. 'This is real life, Jimmy. We are dealing with some of the most vulnerable people in town. They aren't suddenly going to become all happy and motivated. Sometimes just getting them through each day is achievement enough. We live in a broken society, we just have to do our best.'

She paused, and looked me up and down. 'Tell you what, new boy. If you're so keen to stimulate people, I'll let you have a go next year.' She pointed at the office calendar. 'You can try to recruit clients to do gardening, go walking, that sort of thing. I bet it'll be a lot harder than you think.' She frowned. 'You want to work with mentally ill kids, too, huh?' I nodded. 'OK, I'll set you up. And I've got a friend who's a prison nurse. Fancy a placement behind bars?'

'Why not,' I said.

'The harder the strife, Jimmy, the purer the life, that's my motto.' She winked at me. 'You're gonna have one hell of a final year, new boy.'

At the end of term we had a joint lecture with all the different nursing groups. I looked around the Grand Hall. At least a third of the students had dropped out since that opening lecture two years ago. Out of my original children's group, only Vicky, Jana, Hadia and Coco remained, all huddled together at the back. Kiko and the rest of the mental health group had fared better, and lost only four students since the outset. This included a young mother, who'd left temporarily to have a baby, and a trio of others who'd had to retake exams. Only one group had actually increased in numbers – the pigeons. There were now three of them roosting on the ceiling beam.

Super Nurse, with her dazzling smile perfectly in place, made her usual Tiggerish entrance, with Mr Temple stalking moodily behind her. The Doctor and Tanya drew up the rear, representing the mental health department.

Super Nurse kicked off by rallying us with a typically upbeat call to arms: 'This year will be your destiny, students, embrace it!' Mr Temple followed up with his usual gloom fest: 'The last year is always the hardest of all – and don't think you can't fail at this stage. You most certainly can!' He finished off by throwing his Biro at the pigeons, and promising that next time he'd bring a shotgun.

Before we headed off, The Doctor and Tanya took the mental health group to one side. They emphasised that in the third year we could choose our own placements, but it was vital we clocked up the necessary number of working hours. I still had around 850 hours to go.

'And remember you have the drug exam soon,' said Tanya. She waved a book called *Drug Calculations for Student Nurses* over her head. 'Read this, my dears. Cover to cover. And practise drug calculations on all your placements. You need 100 per cent. Full Monty. Nintey-nine per cent won't cut it. You'll fail.'

'And think about what happens when you qualify,' said The Doctor, smoothing his jacket. 'You need to start preparing your CVs. Mental illness is a wide arena. Think how you can best serve it.'

We dispersed and wished each other a happy summer – we had three weeks off. As we embraced, high-fived or shook hands, I realised how little I had got to know this group outside of lectures. Other than regular banter with Kiko and the odd coffee with Nina, Nicola and Joe, we'd spent much of our time away from each other, in hospitals, the community or writing essays.

It was my old group whom I always tended to gravitate back to. The first year was like a distant memory now. We had so much time back then: time to put the world to rights over drinks; time for military fitness, curry nights, each other. Sure, there had been exams, CPR, blood pressures, ward work, but it had been far from all-consuming. In the second year, though, free time had been precious and in the third year was likely to erode completely.

After the lecture I'd agreed to meet with Jana at a local cafe to celebrate surviving the course so far. Despite wearing her normal flamboyant garb – a red beret and an Oasis T-shirt – she seemed in a sullen mood, and sat in silence as I banged on about my petty concerns: the fact that we mental health nurses couldn't do more to empower patients. Blah, blah. All the stuff I'd already had a beef about with BB.

'Maybe I should have stuck with children's nursing,' I said. 'Its outcomes were more definite. But at least I can do some children's mental health next year . . . '

'I understand your concerns, Jimmy,' Jana said, blowing on her coffee.

What had Jana just said? I understand your concerns! This was not the Jana I knew. Something was seriously up with her. I had wanted to meet because she was good at telling me to get a grip. But she was unnaturally placid today. She hadn't been herself when we'd last met at Seamus's pub, but I thought that was just a blip. I was really worried now.

'Jana,' I said. 'You're suspiciously calm. What's up?'

'I think I'm going to quit,' she said softly.

'What!'

'*Sshhh*, Jimmy, don't shout. You heard me.'

'You can't quit, Jana.' I spluttered into my espresso. 'You've reached the third year, you just can't.'

'My last placement was dire, Jimmy. My mentor was a muppet. Horrible to me, and dismissive towards the patients.'

'But that's just one ward.'

'It's the last two, actually.' She paused, staring hard at the table. 'And I've got this job on the side.'

'Not Starbucks, I hope.'

'No, it's a clothes shop. I've been making decent money. It's so good to earn a wage again.' She rapped her hand on the table. 'Dammit, Jimmy, I'm thirty now. I want to settle down, have kids. How can I do that as a nurse? It's so fucking stressful. The hours are long, the pay is pants. I loved the first year, I was so full of hope, but recently I've felt so isolated, so bogged down.

Ward, essay, ward, essay! That's my life. And the nursing hall's such a dump. The girl next door found a mouse in her room yesterday . . . '

'Woahh, Jana,' I urged. 'Come on, you can move out of the hall. Listen, if ever you are stressed call one of us. Call Vicky or me. Share it, have a drink. You can do this. I've seen you, you're a great nurse. You've got the best grades of all of us.'

'Who cares about that? I'm such a ditz. I thought nursing would be all exciting and interesting, but sometimes it's so mundane. It's hardly *ER* is it? Or even *Holby City*.'

'Don't knock *Holby City*.'

'Seriously, Jimmy.' Jana was in full rant now. 'I wanted a job with camaraderie. Making a difference. We seem to shoot from placement to placement. We all talk about qualifying, this magic bit of paper, but so what? Then we've just got decades more of the same thing. Bullshit politics, long hours, no money. Working in a shop is uninspiring, but at least it doesn't drain you emotionally. I like nursing children but sometimes it's all just too much . . . '

'Jana, listen to me.' I thumped down my cup like a gavel. 'This is all about your mentors. You've had two shitty ones and it's squashed your confidence. Once you have a good one again, all this will change. You've been so revved up in the past. You have to see this through. I want to graduate with you, Jana, so do all the others. One more year, that's all, then you can pick your own ward . . . '

'If there's any jobs . . . '

'Of course there'll be jobs, you're the top student in our group! And, hey, how are you ever going to marry a doctor if you work in a clothes shop? You're going to be fine. Trust me on this.' I gave her my best earnest look. 'I'm a mental health nurse.'

Jana smiled. 'Mr Temple won't be very happy if I go, will he?'

'He most certainly won't! And how can you possibly let

Mr T down?' I held out my hand. 'Jana, promise me you won't quit. I want you to shake on it. And if ever you have doubts, promise you'll call me.'

Jana looked me in the eye. 'Yes, sir. Captain Military Fitness.' She straightened her beret and saluted. 'I want to graduate with you, too.' She shook my hand and sighed. 'One more year, Jimmy. One more year.'

Chapter 13

CLUNK

As BB promised, the third year started with a bang – on day one she had enrolled us both in a self-defence course run by Barry, a pumped-up, moustachioed bruiser dressed in a white kung fu suit.

Including BB and myself there were a dozen of us in the class – a mix of therapists, nurses and a wild-bearded American pastor called Blair. We all needed to undergo Barry's initiation as each of us – with the exception of BB – was soon to spend some time working in prison. BB just thought the course would be useful: 'I live in a rough area, new boy!'

Barry clapped his hands to get our attention. We gathered around him, all of us barefoot on the blue matting, surrounded by posters of Bruce Lee and Steven Seagal striking manly poses. Barry started by telling us the difference between being attacked by a woman or by a man.

'So when a lady comes at you,' he explained to his assembled students, 'she's likely to be holding a weapon above her head.'

Barry demonstrated by raising his fist high in the air and bringing it down on my ribcage. Despite my stab-proof vest I teetered and fell over backwards. I gave Barry a steely glare.

'At least I didn't hit you in the wangers, hey, Jimmy,' said

Barry. *Wangers?* He pointed at his groin and roared with laughter. He then winked at one of the other students, Clarissa, a graceful psychotherapist who looked like a hippy version of Kristin Scott Thomas. She wore bell-bottoms, braids in her hair and a T-shirt that read: BLESSED ARE THE CRACKED, FOR THEY LET IN THE LIGHT.

Having recovered from Barry's initial punch I staggered back to my feet. Barry continued his lecture, explaining that men, unlike women, tend to attack low and hit upwards into the chest.

'Like this!' he said, boxing me even more vigorously than the first time. Despite bracing myself, I landed flat on my back. 'Ouch,' I said. This was no fun: it made Military Fitness look like a Pilates class. I was beginning to take Barry's punches personally.

'Jimmy's been felled twice now,' said Barry. 'We can't have that, can we? So let's learn how to defend ourselves.'

Barry pointed out some of the body's more vulnerable regions and soon after, once we had encased ourselves in more protective padding, he ordered us to beat seven bells out of each other.

BB and I partnered up. She looked even more terrifying than normal, her eyes agog, her hair a wild frizz of black. Imagine Ann Widdecombe zapped by a lightning bolt. Barry had given her free rein to stamp on my shins, bash my chest or 'gingerly' knee my groin. Sadly, the word 'gingerly' was not part of BB's vocabulary. Every time she laid into me, I felt my testicles flinch.

While performing a number of manoeuvres on me BB had to shout at the top of her voice 'Get back!', at the same time pushing herself away from me and extricating herself from danger.

'Your turn to come at me now, new boy,' BB said, after pummelling me for a few minutes. She strapped on her protective gear. 'But hurt me and I'll kill you.'

While facing up to BB, I looked across at Clarissa. She was punching Barry's impenetrable six-pack as hard as she could, clearly wowed by his machismo.

'I don't want to hurt you,' said Clarissa.

'Don't worry, sweetpea,' said Barry, eyes locked on her cleavage. 'I used to box when I was younger. Never lost a fight. Takes a lot to hurt me.'

He made it sound as if he was sparring with Rocky Balboa, not an eight-stone hippy chick with fists like wool.

'All right, that's enough now, everyone,' shouted Barry, raising his hands in the air. 'Over here, please. I have something important to say.' He clapped for silence. 'I want to stress physical restraint is used only as an absolute last resort. Verbal de-escalation is always best. Got that?' He paused, looking over to Clarissa for approval. 'As the great Winston Churchill once said: "To jaw, jaw is always better than to war, war".'

Clarissa nodded in agreement and eagerly applauded. I hoped she was clapping Churchill rather than Barry. She clearly thought our boastful instructor was the bee's knees, poor girl.

To round off the session we watched Barry wrest himself into some sort of ultra-protective silver suit. It looked so impregnable even a cruise missile wouldn't dent it, let alone a bunch of slack-biceped therapists, nurses and holy men.

'That suit makes you look a bit like a superhero, Barry,' said Clarissa.

'More like a ponce in cling film,' I suggested.

Actually I didn't. Barry was quite a lot bigger than me, and knew how to kill people with his thumbs. Even if I had a Kalashnikov and he had both hands tied behind his back, I'd still put my money on him.

'Right, everyone,' said Barry, puffing out his chest. 'I want you to form a circle around me and take it in turns to charge at me. Do your worst. Hit me in the stomach, kick my shins, go for my groin.' He winked at Clarissa. Honestly, the man had all the sexual nuances of a baboon. 'Do whatever you want to me. I can handle it.'

Yes, you tosspot, so could any of us 'handle it' if we were clad in a suit of kryptonite, or whatever super-strength fibre he was sporting.

'Go!' shouted Barry. 'Do your worst!' We all took it in turns to charge at him – knee, kick, punch – and then shout 'Get back!' as we pushed ourselves away. I went in as hard as I could, but failed to make much impact, ricocheting off Barry's suit into a nearby punchbag. Barry was whipping us into a state of fury. By far the most violent member of the class, other than BB, was Blair, the newly appointed prison pastor. He threw himself at Barry like some sort of rabid crusader.

'Come on, you lot,' goaded Barry. 'I can hardly feel a thing. Give me all you've got.'

We all continued to slog away at him until Clarissa, whose punches normally had all the power of a puffball, accidentally hit Barry on the nose – the one part of his body that wasn't protected.

'Arghh,' shouted Barry, clutching his face.

'Good shot, girlfriend!' whispered BB.

'Oh, I'm so sorry,' said Clarissa, running up to Barry. 'My punch bounced off your suit.'

'Arghh,' said Barry. He really wasn't being very stoic about it. A drop of his blood spilled on to the dojo floor.

'I'm a nurse, let me take a look,' said BB, motioning for Barry to sit down. 'Looks like you taught Clarissa to punch well.' BB nodded at me. 'Bring me some tissues will you, Jimmy.' I dashed to get some, and watched as BB nursed the whimpering Barry. 'Come on, big man,' she urged. 'Your nose isn't broken, only a little knock.'

'Arghh,' said Barry.

The class had definitely been worth it. I not only knew what to do if confronted by an aggressive prisoner, I'd further had the joy of watching Clarissa deck beefcake Barry. It was a scene to gladden the hardest of hearts. A modern-day David and Goliath, only better, as our Goliath had on a kryptonite suit.

'So Clarissa found Barry's Achilles' heel,' I said to BB, as we made our way back to the office. We both hooted with laughter, showing a worrying lack of unconditional positive regard towards our bruised instructor.

'Forget his heel,' said BB. 'Clarissa found his Barry's Nose. That's a far better expression.' She turned to me, suddenly serious. 'I've never asked you about your Barry's Nose, new boy. Other than your taste in shirts.'

'Well, I once injured my hamstring . . . '

'I don't mean your physical Barry's Nose,' she interrupted. 'I mean what's your deepest mental vulnerability? Your deepest prejudice? What are your demons?' BB tapped her head. 'The things you are outwardly confident about, but deep down terrify you?'

'Wow, BB, that's a bit heavy.'

'Not really,' she said. 'I'm your mentor and should know these things. You don't have to tell me, of course, but it's not a bad idea. You are dealing with mentally unwell people on a daily basis, Jimmy. To treat them successfully you need to know your own fears and be prepared to accept them.' She smiled. 'Just have a think about it, that's all.'

'OK, I'll do that,' I told her. After a pause I added: 'My current big fear is very obvious.'

'What's that?'

'Starting my prison placement next week.'

CLUNK! CLANG! CLINK! It's hard to describe exactly the noise a prison door makes when it slams shut. I found its metallic echo a bit sinister; there was a horrid finality to it. Of course, for me the sound only meant I was locked in for the duration of my shift. For the prisoners it could mean this was home for months, years or, in rare cases, decades.

But to Mr T (not to be confused with Mr Temple), the avuncular prison officer escorting me to my new ward, it was a comforting sound.

'I just love that clunk!' he told me as we walked through a yard of exercising prisoners. 'Something reassuring about it.' At first I put his observation on a par with the loopy general in *Apocalypse Now* who loves 'the smell of napalm in the morning', but by the end of my month in the prison I could understand what he meant.

I'd already handed in my mobile phone at reception – it was 100 per cent forbidden to have them on the premises in case they got into a prisoner's hands. I had no problem with this. In fact I relished escaping my mobile's pervasive trills whenever possible. I'd also signed in at the door, shown my ID and explained I was a student nurse.

'Blimey,' said the prison receptionist, pinning a pass to my jumper. 'We don't get many of them.'

I was to be based on a mental health ward within the prison. Prisoners in general are known to have disproportionately high rates of mental illness, and this prison was no exception, with several of the inmates self-harming, and up to 80 per cent battling drink and drug problems.

Soon I was standing in the ward's station, trying not to look nervous. The room was divided in two with a big communal table in the middle. It resembled a teacher's common room – except for a pair of handcuffs hanging from a chair. The prison officers were on one side and the nurses on the other.

A prison officer, straight out of central casting, walked over to me. He was a dead ringer for Ross Kemp with a 'who the hell are you' look on his face.

'Here, have some tea, mate.' The officer's face lit up with a smile, and he handed me a cup. 'Welcome to the team.' Seconds later a nurse offered me a biscuit. I immediately relaxed – this is going to be all right, I thought. I'd noticed over the last couple of years that the more high-security a placement, the friendlier the staff. A lazy generalisation, maybe, but in this place it rang true.

The assembled prison officers (all in dark uniforms) and nurses (the smartest looking mental health nurses I'd seen to date) all listened to the handover, presented by a tired-looking night shift nurse. In hangdog tones she revealed that of the fifteen prisoners, all female, one had self-harmed that night by tying a ligature around her neck. Another had carried out a 'dirty protest', spreading urine and faeces all over her cell walls, and another was convinced she was the Queen. This all sounded pretty serious to me, but none of the officers or nurses batted an eyelid.

After the handover I met my mentor, a jovial Nigerian with a booming voice and a penchant for hearty backslaps. I nicknamed him Pickwick. He took me to one side to give me the low-down. The first thing he pointed out was that he and I had to hit it off.

'We'll be as good as handcuffed together, Jimmy,' Pickwick explained. 'As a student you're not allowed prison keys. Someone's got to go everywhere with you to unlock doors – even when you take a piss.'

The prison in question was London's Holloway, the largest women's jail in Europe, holding up to 500 inmates. I'd learnt this from a fact sheet presented to me by Pickwick. Other interesting nuggets revealed that Holloway, after years as a mixed prison, became women-only in 1902. Over time the prison has locked away everyone from blue-blooded suffragettes to cold-blooded killers, including Myra Hindley. Ruth Ellis, the last woman to be executed in Britain, was hanged at Holloway in 1955.

Holloway was not in my usual neck of the woods, so I travelled into north London at the start of each week. Kiko had requested his 'elective' at Pentonville Prison (only a short walk from Holloway) thinking that the work might suit him, too.

I spent my first days helping with medication rounds, keeping watch on any self-harmers, or joining in activity workshops with the prisoners. Some of the women were withdrawn, some charming, and some in-your-face troublemakers, constantly hurling abuse or demanding things. On my first shift I had to refuse to reveal my mobile number and family details on an hourly basis.

Pickwick told me it was vital to keep my private life under wraps. This was in case a patient tried to track me down after she was released. It had happened only recently with a nurse from a male prison. An inmate had turned up at the nurse's family home only hours after being set free, having followed her on a bus. This particular prisoner had purely been lonely and no harm was caused, but if he had been aggressive or vindictive things might well have turned nasty.

This same 'no private life' rule always applied on mental health wards, but in prisons special vigilance was needed. Prison officers were especially careful, in case any prisoners had built up a grudge about being restrained or disciplined during their stay.

One big difference at Holloway, compared to my other placements, was having the nurses work alongside the prison officers. It amused me that the officers were never called by their first names. They were all referred to as 'Sir', 'Maam' or by their surname, 'Mr Smith', 'Mrs Jones' – it sounded part *Porridge*, part *Reservoir Dogs*. Nurses, though, were just called 'Jimmy' or 'Florence', and were far fewer in number.

This made sense. Unlike on my previous wards, here it was the prison officers not the nurses who dealt with any incidents of control or restraint. The officers also mopped up any 'dirty protests' (I was delighted to learn this) and generally took care of ward discipline. This left the nurses to do what they did best, the caring side of things.

During my first week an argument sprang up between the nurses and prison officers as to whether the women on our ward should be called 'prisoners' or 'patients'. After many passionate exchanges – 'Prisoners are still human beings, you know,' Pickwick might say, to which Mr T would respond: 'Of course, prisoners are human beings, what else would they be, wombats?' – it was agreed that prison officers preferred to call them 'prisoners', and nurses 'patients'. I'd heard the dynamic between officers and nurses could be tense. On this ward, it was pretty harmonious, the officers being firm but fair types who made every effort to build up a good rapport with their prisoners.

But I'd be lying if I said I didn't find the first week tough. Many of the women came to the ward from incredibly harsh backgrounds, with around 50 per cent of them having been abused. It was to the prison's credit that its last suicide had been almost a year earlier, although several women admitted they had attempted suicide and many others had self-harmed. Their stories were often grim beyond belief.

'There's lots of bragging and bad behaviour here,' said Pickwick. 'Some of the women call it Hotel Holloway as if it's a soft touch. But that's just bravado, a way to cope. There's also lots of sadness and vulnerability, especially on the mental health wards. But for some girls it really is a safe haven. Their life is so hard on the outside, that prison is preferable.'

I met up for a pint with Kiko on Friday evening after we'd both completed our second week behind bars. Kiko was clearly loving it.

'The team are great, very professional,' said Kiko. 'It's the best place I've worked so far. Can't believe the size of the prison though, over a thousand prisoners.'

Kiko said Pentonville was known as the locals' prison. Unlike Holloway, the lion's share of the inmates came from north London, many of them 'druggies or thieves'. Everyone from Oscar Wilde to Pete Doherty had been banged up there.

'There's a high turnover,' said Kiko. 'Some stay only a few days, but they might well be back again.' He picked at his beer mat pensively. 'On the mental health ward I'm at there's a few long-term patients, though. Some have severe personality disorders and they'd struggle on the outside.'

I knew that at Holloway the average stay of an inmate was only forty-five days, but it wasn't encouraging to learn that, nationally, over 60 per cent of women released from prisons were back behind bars within two years. I'd also read somewhere that Britain, proportionate to its national population, had one of the highest number of prisoners Europe.

'Is it scary in a men's prison?' I asked Kiko.

'Not really,' he said. 'I was threatened a couple of times, but nothing too bad. Just testing me out. One of the officers told me he'd been stabbed with a pen once. But the team are very slick at dealing with any aggro.' Kiko smiled. 'Sometimes I reckon prison officers, for all their toughness, have to be more compassionate than us nurses.'

I remember Pickwick had told me he'd worked in both men's and women's jails. He said men tended to threaten violence when stressed, whereas women would be more likely to have emotional outbursts or resort to self-harm.

'So is Holloway anything like that TV show *Bad Girls*?' asked Kiko. 'Any nymphomaniac lesbians?'

'In your dreams, you shallow git,' I replied, grinning. I suspected that comparing a prison officer's life to *Bad Girls* was like comparing a nurse's job to *Casualty* – worlds apart.

But, talking to Kiko, it sounded as if there were many similarities between the two prisons. One thing that struck me was that Holloway was so much more than just a place of correction. Other than mental health wards it had an all-singing, all-dancing detox unit, a remand centre, a homeless refuge, a mother and baby unit, education facilities, a gym and a swimming pool.

'Yeah, Pentonville's pretty good too,' said Kiko. 'They even have a chapel – I said a prayer there on my way out the other day.' He munched ruminatively on a crisp. 'Prisoners can get work, too, you know. They sometimes make money putting the spongy bits on airline headsets. They only get a few quid a day. Still, better than nothing, hey.'

It seemed both of us had been impressed by our individual prison facilities and their staff. Kiko told me his ward had a prison officer who'd worked in France. He'd revealed that France had some of the worst jails in Europe – overcrowded and with poor rehab and mental health facilities. Indeed, the previous year France had lost 115 prisoners to suicide; the UK roughly half that, despite having more prisoners.

'I've heard the worst suicide rates in prison are among the Australian aborigines,' said Kiko. 'I suppose being caged up is the worst thing in the world for nomadic people like them. Hell on earth.'

I pondered this, and decided that despite all the self-harm at Holloway, the fact so few women had committed suicide was a huge achievement.

To break our pensive mood I told Kiko I was due to start work in Holloway's detox unit for a couple of shifts the following week.

'Good luck to you, that's what I say, mate,' said Kiko, draining his pint. 'There's always a few drugs circulating with our prisoners. They hide them everywhere – up their bum, under their foreskin.' I grimaced at this news. 'But officers are getting better at locating them now. Using dogs, detectors, you name it. We've got a good drug rehab unit, too, where dozens of prisoners kick the habit.'

As a nurse I would not be involved in locating drugs, only administering them to detox patients. But as 80 per cent of Holloway's women had drug and alcohol problems, I sensed next week would be a busy one.

'You know, Jimmy,' said Kiko, wistfully. 'I like nursing in a prison. Challenging job, great team spirit, good pension.' His face lit up. 'I think I've found what I want to do.'

As for me, I wasn't so sure.

The next day I was on the prison detox unit, measuring up cup after cup of an emerald-green fluid. This was methadone, a heroin substitute, which does everything heroin does except deliver 'the hit'.

'Methadone's a prescribed drug,' said Pickwick, studying a drug chart next to me. 'Keeps the doctors busy, busy, *busy* scribbling out forms, I can tell you.'

Dozens of patients snaked around the wall to the side of the treatment room. Before taking their dose each of them had to have their blood pressure taken. As methadone acts as an opiate it was important that each patient had a BP high enough to prevent the drug fatally slowing down their system.

We were certainly pouring out methadone at an alarming rate – quicker than pints at a rugby club dinner. Pickwick told me its use in prisons had risen by over 50 per cent in a single year.

'Many women here take methadone every day,' said Pickwick, handing a cup of it to a dull-eyed woman with long, grey hair. 'It stops the craving for heroin. If they successfully detox here they're able to get weekly prescriptions on the outside but only if they can prove they are not using heroin on top.'

Methadone is controversial stuff. Some experts see it as simply a 'liquid cosh' to keep troublesome inmates subdued, while others swear by it, claiming that it helps stabilise addicts' lives, making it easier for them to quit in the long run. One study showed almost half of those treated with methadone gave up drugs within ten months.

'I've seen methadone work wonders,' said Pickwick, pouring out another dose. 'But I also wonder about the logic of substituting one drug for another. And at three to five grand per patient a year it's not cheap. Critics argue that the money should be spent on cancer drugs instead.'

Pickwick added that some experts believe addicts should be allowed to use heroin within the NHS, but only in controlled conditions in special 'shooting galleries' in the community. Some, like Pickwick, believed that this legalised shooting-up would cut deaths by causing fewer dirty needles and less crime. Others, including Mr T, thought it was expensive – PC touchy-feelyness gone wild.*

After administering dozens more cups of methadone, I moved into the neighbouring room. Here Subutex, another heroin substitute, was being administered to the prisoners. It was taken as a tablet placed under the tongue.

'Subutex is an opiate too,' said Pickwick, waving at a prisoner with pink-dyed hair. 'And its dosage can be decreased much quicker – over weeks rather than months. But, one hitch, it's much more expensive.' Pickwick flicked his wrist to demonstrate wasted money. 'Those taking it really need to be ready to quit.'

Pickwick mentioned that occasionally girls deliberately broke the law in order to get into Holloway, purely to detox.

'The detox programme here has a great reputation,' he said. 'But it's sad that young girls have to offend purely to get on it.' He scratched his head distractedly. 'Of course, some addicts are so shot to pieces they only want to get clean so they can inject and feel high again. The community should do more to help these women.' Pickwick grabbed my arm. 'Now let me show you something that will really break your heart.'

Pickwick led me up several flights of stairs, occasionally stopping to unlock barred doorways. We entered a warm, carpeted room with children's drawings decorating the walls. This was

*Peter Carter, the Chief Executive of the Royal College of Nursing, has recently spoken out in favour of shooting galleries for heroin addicts within the NHS.

the reception area to Holloway's mother and baby unit, where we had arranged to meet one of the mothers.

'Over half the women in prisons have a child under sixteen,' said Pickwick, beckoning a young mother over to us. 'And 20 per cent are single mums. Most of the mothers have the tragedy of being separated from their kids while in prison. But . . . ' He smiled at the mother. 'Little babies are allowed to stay here.'

I shook hands with the mother. Her name was Betty, a tiny, stick-thin ex-heroin user, who was now clean thanks to Holloway's detox programme. Betty said she was happy to talk to me – Pickwick had already cleared this. She cut straight to the chase and immediately revealed that her baby son had been a drug addict on the day he was born. Betty lifted up her pallid arm to show me where it had been pockmarked by needles.

'I was shooting-up heroin every day for ages,' said Betty. 'Or if not, I'd smoke crack. Easier to get, and very buzzy. But I always preferred smack – oops. She raised her hand in apology. 'Sorry, love, if you didn't know, smack's just another word for heroin. Anyway, heroin, H, smack, don't matter what it's called, after a couple of years injecting the stuff the veins on my arms were useless. Needed to move on to my legs.'

'The veins in the legs are more dangerous,' said Pickwick. He explained they are nearer the major arteries, which, if hit, could cause fatal bleeding. Long-term use of heroin could also lead to thrombosis and then possible amputation.

'I was a wreck,' added Betty. 'My partner beat me up and kept coming back. Then I got nicked for dealing, once I'd given birth. Coming here and detoxing has changed my life. But I still feel so ashamed . . . '

At this point Betty dissolved in tears, unable to carry on talking. She held her son close, a tiny blue hat covering his face. 'I'm so ashamed,' she said, sobbing wildly. 'So ashamed what I did to my little boy.' She repeated this several times before we decided to leave her in peace.

Pickwick explained that the heroin had crossed Betty's placenta to her son in her womb, leading him to become addicted. But when he'd been born, Betty's heroin was no longer available to him and he'd immediately gone into withdrawal. In a Specialist Care Baby Unit he had been given morphine (taken in drops with his milk) to fight his addiction. He had fortunately pulled through, although it was too early to tell if he had completely avoided any developmental problems. Pickwick said Betty felt genuine remorse and had managed to kick the heroin, something many others failed to do.

'A baby can become addicted to methadone in the womb, too,' said Pickwick as we walked back to our ward. 'It doesn't have to be heroin. Whatever the drug, Jimmy, it's a hell of a tough start to life. Cold turkey from day one.'

I came away that evening reeling. Mr T, as usual, escorted me back to the reception. Before he clunked the door behind us, I asked him why he liked the clunking sound. I'd been wanting to know since my first day.

'Well, for starters that clunk signals the end of a bloody shift – always good in my book,' he said, turning the key. 'You see, Jimmy, when a prison door clunks it means there is a sense of order. Our job is to make sure these women are held safely but also to sort them out, try to get them back in the world again.' He smiled. 'Hopefully they'll appreciate that clunk one day too, when it means they're free.'

I walked away from Holloway and waited at the bus stop opposite the prison gates. From the outside Holloway didn't look like a prison at all, tucked away amid terraced houses; a pub and petrol station diagonally opposite. It looked more like a railway station or an old school. I even knew the area a little bit as my sister lived nearby. I'd probably even walked past it a few times without once questioning its purpose.

211

Well, now Holloway had yielded just a few of its secrets to me, and I was grateful for that. I knew I didn't want to work in a prison – it wasn't really for me, and I probably wasn't tough enough – but, thanks to Pickwick, Mr T and the team, the clunk of its gates seemed far less sinister, and the women behind them far more human.

That evening I received an email from Kay in Mexico:

Jimmy!

I'm setting up a street child project early next year with some Mexican colleagues. Are you still interested? You, me and Jack always talked of something like this. He's already said no – too loved up with his señorita. I know it's a long shot for you, Jimmy, but let me know if you still want to volunteer for a while. Any time you can spare at the beginning would be great. Just on the off-chance, hombre!

Hasta luego,

Kay x

I wished my friend luck, and reluctantly told her that I'd be unable to join her.

Chapter 14

BARRY'S NOSE

A week later I was released from prison and posted back to the community with BB. This gave me a chance to see some old faces – Joanna, Leanne, Raj – to practise more depot injections and meet some fresh clients.

One client that made a big impression during this time was an ex-soldier called Bert. I knew some ex-servicemen were vulnerable to mental illness but Bert was the first one to cross my path. He had recently been admitted on an acute ward after causing mayhem in a public park, swigging whisky and shouting abuse at passersby. BB knew Bert well and was particularly keen for me to work with him.

Bert's ward was dingy and crowded, with a TV blasting out sugary pop tunes. The other clients all looked defeated or spaced out, with Bert an animated exception. BB sought out a quiet area near the nurses' station. She chatted to Bert for a while and then suggested I speak to him alone while she visited another of her clients in a neighbouring ward.

BB had already filled me in quite a bit about Bert. I knew that he had served in his regiment, the Green Jackets, for over a decade and fought in the first Iraq war. He left the army in the late 1990s to set up a cleaning business with his girlfriend, but civvy street never suited him.

'I missed the army so much,' Bert told me, rubbing his silvery stubble. 'My mates, the banter, the hint of danger. I was good at being a soldier. Bloody good.' He nodded his head. 'But out of uniform I was hopeless. Got pissed up the whole time, shouted at my girl. Our business didn't stand a chance. She kicked me out.'

As a palliative to his wounded pride, Bert backpacked the world, funded by his remaining savings. He trekked in the Himalayas, jitterbugged through Indo-China and worked on cattle stations in Australia. He enjoyed it, but felt very lonely. When he arrived in America he'd almost run out of money. He tried hitch-hiking from California to New York but nobody wanted to pick him up.

'I must have looked well dodgy,' conceded Bert, laughing. 'No one wants to pick up a man in his forties with a shaved head and Bermuda shorts.'

'I usually pick up hitch-hikers,' I said. 'But, you're right, I'd draw the line at that.'

After his travels Bert flew back to London, penniless, his confidence in freefall. His parents were dead; his sister didn't speak to him. He relied on the kindness of a couple of childhood friends, but knew they could only carry him for so long.

'People ask me why I didn't just knuckle down,' said Bert. 'But it's tough sleeping on floors, hard to get your shit together. I was too proud to ask for help. To get benefits you have to fill in loads of forms. I was a soldier, not a secretary.'

Bert paused to sip on his coffee. He took off his jumper and stretched. I noticed SUZIE tattooed on his bicep. He told me it was his ex-girlfriend's name, the one who'd wanted to set up a cleaning business. There hadn't been any girlfriends since ('No woman wants a tramp, mate, but I really miss the sex'). He leant forward pensively, resting his jowls on his palms.

'I can't believe how this happened to me,' he mused. 'How I pissed it all away.' He nudged my shoulder. 'But trust me, mate, anyone can end up on the street.'

According to Bert, the days of the homeless all being dropouts and wasters were long gone. Take him, a proud ex-serviceman, isolated after all the camaraderie of army life, or any number of others in the armed forces suffering mental illness (post-traumatic stress disorder, depression) after serving in Iraq and Afghanistan.

'I tried to top myself about a year ago,' Bert confided. 'I was just so alone, nothing to live for, depressed as hell. I ate a stack of Paracetamol washed down with a bottle of rum.' He smiled sadly. 'I woke up in A & E with a mother, son and a Holy Ghost of a headache. That's when I first met BB. She's helped a lot. She even got me some electroconvulsive therapy.' He jabbed a finger into his forehead to demonstrate. 'It gets a bad rap because of all those movies with folks getting their brains fried, but it can be really good. Definitely picked me up a bit.'

BB had also contacted one of Bert's old army mates who'd agreed to put him up in a spare room. Bert explained that the homeless often have some sort of shelter – with a friend, a parent – but anyone with no shelter is called a 'rough sleeper'. According to the government there were currently fewer than 500 rough sleepers in the whole country – a figure Bert considered 'bollocks' and far too low.

'I'm lucky my army pal's been so generous,' said Bert, rolling a cigarette. 'Him and his family have been so great.' His voice cracked at this point. 'But sometimes, mate, I really need a blowout, go back to sleeping rough. Get smashed. It's hard to understand, but there's a sort of solidarity on the street. I need to be around people as fucked up as me, got nothing to prove to them.'

Bert cheered as BB came back. He told me that BB was his heroine and had recently been trying to get him into a hostel for ex-soldiers.

'It would be great to be among soldiers again,' Bert mused. 'But I'm still worried about feeling a failure, a drain on society.'

'You served your country, for God's sake!' BB said, shaking a fist at him. 'You were willing to lay down your life. That's more than most of us ever do. You deserve help.'

'That feels like another lifetime away, BB.' Bert kicked at the floor. 'I look at the pictures of me in uniform and it's like I'm a different man. My life had some meaning. But now I'm all messed up.' He winked at me. 'Now, my friend, I'm three stops short of Dagenham.'

'Three stops short of Dagenham?' I asked.

Bert roared with laughter. 'Barking, mate,' he said. 'I'm fucking barking.'

I liked Bert and continued to visit him over the following weeks. I wanted him to be one of the clients I would 'stimulate' (as BB cynically put it) with activities such as gardening, sport or music.

To start with I encouraged Bert to attend the team's weekly social drop-ins. These were simple knees-ups in a local community centre providing hot drinks, snacks and a chance for clients to chat. The attendance was usually poor, rarely breaking double figures, but at least those who did come seemed to enjoy it.

At one drop-in I tried to rustle up volunteers to do some gardening work run by a local mental health charity. Several clients expressed interest but when push came to shove only Bert and Leanne turned up. That morning Bert hacked down nettles with a sickle while Leanne weeded a flower bed. They both loved it but later I apologised to BB for managing to recruit only the two of them.

'Don't be sorry, new boy,' said BB. 'It's a result to get anybody. Just don't be disappointed if they don't keep it up.'

Sure enough, despite assuring me that they would both garden the following week, only Bert made it. Leanne felt too tired. The week after only Leanne made it: Bert was ill. And so it went on. Yet for all their inconsistency, the gardening clearly gave

Bert and Leanne a huge confidence boost every time they did it, and I was heartened by this.

One other client I was particularly keen to get along to the gardening was Carly who was only twenty, one of the youngest on our team's books. She was in a wretched situation, clinically depressed and dependent on drink. She never left her mother's flat, afraid even to go to the local shops. She spent much of her time lying in bed with her cat, watching horribly violent DVDs and swigging vodka. She looked very sick, with jaundiced skin, shaking hands and puffy, pale blue-eyes.

Carly's flat was often full of her alcoholic mother's seedy-looking friends. Carly never mixed with people her own age, and the mother never encouraged her to. Her mother enjoyed having Carly at her beck and call, plus the state handouts that came with having a mentally unwell daughter. There was little our team could do to change the situation. Apart from her self-destructive lifestyle, the mother was not abusing Carly, and her daughter seemed devoted to her.

I saw Carly regularly over the following weeks. Every time I asked her if she'd like to do something with the team – 'What about a walk in the park, Carly? Gardening? The zoo?' – she always blanked me. I was about to give up, when one day she told me she'd like to visit the cinema. I wasn't sure if this would be seen as a constructive activity but BB was more than happy for us to go. 'Do it, new boy, anything at all that sparks her interest.' Carly's mother predictably tried to prevent the trip, saying Carly wouldn't be able to cope, but BB persuaded her it would be fine.

So, one evening, Carly, Raj (wearing my gay cowboy shirt), Bert and Leanne all gathered for a visit to the local cinema with BB and myself. It wasn't plain sailing at all. Carly had a panic attack on the bus, Leanne spilt takeaway pizza all down her front, and Bert got angry with someone who trod on his toe. Due to Leanne spending twenty minutes dolling herself up in the cinema toilet we missed the first part of the film – *Slumdog Millionaire* – but on the whole the trip was a success. Carly enjoyed it so much she even demonstrated some Bollywood dancing back at her flat.

I continued to take small groups of clients – always with BB or another nurse – to various activities. Sometimes the clients turned up, sometimes they didn't. Being a student I had the flexibility to organise these trips, but soon it was time for me to start my other placements. I had exams looming, too. I was gutted to let these group activities slip, especially as BB and the team had no time to continue them.

I told BB she was right. I hadn't made as much impact as I'd hoped with my 'stimulating' activities, and had only press-ganged a very small posse of clients.

'Yeah, waste of time, new boy,' said BB, all matter of fact. She carried on writing her notes. I felt shell-shocked.

'Oh, you're such a sucker, Jimmy!' BB smiled and walked over to me. 'You did much better than I thought you would. Getting Carly out of her flat was a coup. You did stuff we have no time for.' She shook my shoulders. 'That's what a student should do. Shake up their mentors a bit. We get very programmed into what we do – medication, care plans. Blah, blah. We get cynical. Yes, you can be a fool, Jimmy – a hopelessly idealistic, naive, pedantic, sartorially disastrous pain in the butt, but you did OK. Take that as a compliment.'

'That was a compliment!'

'Jesus, new boy, what do you want me to do? Pop the champagne! Fire twenty-one guns! Get the Red Arrows to do a fly past! You did OK. Now get out of here.' I walked towards the door. 'Oh, one other bit of good news. You'll be glad to hear Bert has been accepted into a rehab centre for ex-servicemen. He's over the moon. Moving in next week. All your sodding stimulation might have done him some good after all.'

That night I got a call from Hadia. Next placement she would be on the same ward as me – one that specialised in children's mental health. In the third year children's nurses were allowed to pick one placement in an area they didn't normally work. I asked her why on earth she'd chosen mentally unwell adolescents.

'No one's called me a fat bitch recently,' said Hadia. I flash-backed to her incident with Mr Smith. 'I thought I'd better toughen myself up again.'

'Good on you,' I replied. 'I look forward to catching up. Mr Temple will be proud of you.'

Hadia cleared her throat. 'I also wanted to ask if you'd heard from Jana, Jimmy? I've been on placement with her and she hasn't turned up for the last few days. She seems to have gone AWOL.'

I called Jana later that evening but got her answering machine. I left her a message. The following day I had a text back: 'Don't panic, old boy, I'm fine. Just doing some thinking.'

I left her to her thoughts – a decision I later came to regret.

The following day in the community with BB I had a power-ful wake-up call. I had gone to visit Raj at his hostel to try to persuade him to join one last gardening trip. He had been very reclusive recently and I hoped to bring him out of his shell.

BB allowed me to visit clients by myself but only if they were in an environment with mental health professionals at hand. Raj's hostel was such a place.

In the past I had always visited Raj with another nurse or social worker, but that particular afternoon I decided I knew him well enough to see him on my own. He was usually so placid and taciturn, I saw no reason to worry.

On arrival at the hostel, the reception was empty. I saw Raj in the sitting room and explained to one of the cleaning ladies who was wiping the windows – I knew all the staff well – that I was going to have a session with him. She waved for me to go ahead and left the room.

I greeted Raj, turned down the TV and sat myself down on a chair at the far end of the room, furthest from the door, which I had closed.

Raj was wearing my purple shirt and rubbing at his patchy, newly grown beard. He looked awful: gaunt and morose.

'How have you been, Raj?' I asked. There was a long pause and I repeated the question.

'Fuck off!' he shouted at me in his thick Indian accent, thrashing his hands down on the sofa. 'Fuck off! Fuck off! Fuck off!' He looked at me with fierce, dilated eyes.

I realised I'd made a colossal error of judgement. I hadn't asked any of the nurses how Raj had been that week. I'd put myself alone in a room with him and shut the door. I'd completely let down my guard.

I tried to placate Raj but he was distraught. Whenever I got up he pointed at me and repeated: 'Fuck off, fuck off . . . ' I had never heard Raj swear before, let alone raise his voice. He'd always seemed one of the most gentle clients, at times anxious but never violent.

After a while he looked away from me, and turned his attention back to the TV. *Countdown* was on, a ticking clock just about audible in the background. Raj seemed transfixed by the screen. I wondered whether to just wait until someone came into the room, and then move, or head for the door.

I inched off my chair. 'Fuck off!' Raj's head swirled round and he pointed at me aggressively. 'Fuck off!' He looked back at the TV, but his insults were definitely addressed at me, not Carol Vorderman. I sat back down again. This was getting awkward. I kicked myself for not following procedure.

Fortunately Jim, one of the hostel nurses, came in after a few minutes. Raj continued to swear and hit the sofa but remained seated. I was able to make my retreat.

Back in the hostel office I learnt that Raj had been playing up all week. It was the anniversary of the death of the old lady he had been so close to. He had covered his shrine to her in his room with flowers and cried a lot. He'd been refusing his medication and often shouting to himself.

My actions while seeing Raj had been incredibly stupid and I didn't really need anyone to tell me so – although BB did, quite forcefully.

'You've started to treat some clients too much like friends, Jimmy,' she insisted. 'Don't ever, ever do that again. Raj has schizophrenia. That means he can be radically different one day to the next. You knew that but you barged in as if he was your best mate. What if he'd attacked you? I've given you a free rein because you're generally quite sensible. Today you were stupid beyond belief. A complete shithead, to be honest.'

And she was right. Because of my trips to gardening groups, parks and the cinema with various clients – Raj, Bert, Leanne, Carly – I believed I had got to know them all well. This, combined with my swelling experience now that I was in my third year, had made me far more confident than I should have been. I had blurred the boundaries between client and nurse. More worryingly, I had forgotten I was still just a student. I had shown a gross error of judgement and acted as BB so eloquently put it: 'like a complete shithead'.

On the final day of my community placement I was sitting on the top deck of a bus with BB. We had just finished doing a series of visits, including one to see Bert, who had now settled in well at his new home.

The air on the bus's top deck was so warm and heavy you could chew it. Everyone was sweating and BB was fanning herself with her hat.

'Look at that, new boy.' BB pointed to a poster advertising for teachers. It depicted a group of cherubic children, smiley and attentive, in front of a teacher who looked like Cheryl Cole. It said something like: *Do Something Wonderful Today – Teach!*

'If that's what teaching is really like,' said BB, chuckling to herself, 'then I'm the Dalai Lama.'

I'd never seen a similar advert for nurses. Perhaps the country was more in need of teachers than nurses at the moment. But what would a nurse advertisement look like? I mused. I doubt the budget would stretch to hiring a Cheryl Cole lookalike. Instead, I imagined a grainy photo of BB with a big syringe and the slogan: *Do Something Wonderful Today – Inject!* Or Mr Temple with a Lord Kitchener moustache, his finger pointing out in an accusatory manner: '*Nurses – You are Mine*'.

I was snapped out of my reverie by the thrum of a ghetto blaster. Two boys in their mid- to late-teens – one black, one white – slumped down in the seats in front of BB and me. The music was horrible – loud, repetitive and fused with violence. The boys talked in boastful voices about a recent fight they'd had, the word 'motherfucker' cropping up regularly. They seemed to have no spatial awareness at all. I noticed there were two elderly ladies sitting directly in front of them, and a young girl of around ten, to their side.

'I think I ought to say something,' I whispered to BB.

She shook her head vehemently. 'Please don't, Jimmy.' BB had an unusual look on her face. One I'd never seen on her before. Then I realised why: she looked scared.

A ladybird flew on to the window beside the white boy with the ghetto blaster. He had a shaved head, as did his black friend. The black boy was playing on a Nintendo, a game with a gothic backdrop and lots of hairy warriors slaughtering each other.

'Fucking ladybug,' shouted the white boy, pointing at the ladybird on the window. 'I'm gonna roast you, motherfucker.'

He handed the ghetto blaster to his friend, fumbled in his pocket and drew out a cigarette lighter. He put the lighter under the ladybird and fired it up. 'Roast, ladybug, yeehaa!' The bug took off and landed on the window next to me. To my horror the boy leaned over, ignoring me completely and started to try to flambé the little insect once again.

'Stop, please!' I said, putting my hand over the ladybird. 'You don't need to burn it.' And then more tentatively, 'your behaviour will scare people. Your swearing, your music. There's children and elderly people on board . . .'

The boy gave me a look of such hatred, I dried up. To my shame I felt scared. Both the boys were in their late-teens but they looked considerably stronger than me. More than that, they seemed fearless, possibly high on something. Since starting my community placement a couple of months earlier I'd been on several buses with teenagers running wild. One time the driver stopped the bus and called the police, causing the troublemakers to scarper. On this bus, the driver was out of eyeshot.

'You don't tell me what to do, OK?' said the white boy, pointing his lighter at me. 'I do what I like. OK!'

His black friend leaned over towards me. His voice was soft and sarcastic. 'Ah, he's all sensitive this man. Doesn't want us to hurt the little ladybug. Ahhh!' The white boy started to laugh. I looked across at BB; her face was uncharacteristically tight and pallid. She remained silent. The bus was half full but everyone seemed to be ignoring our little drama, looking straight ahead. There were several other adults, including a few physically strong men, who could hear every word. No one chose to intervene.

I wanted to scream at all of them, ask them what sort of example this was setting – all of us just sitting there like lemons. Had none of us any self-respect? What about the dignity of the poor ten-year-old and the elderly women? What about the swearing, the vile music, the shameless attitude? Did nobody have a problem with it? I continued to stare at the two boys, but felt impotent and furious.

'What you fucking looking at us like that for, mister?' said the white boy. 'You want to fight or something?'

'Yeah, you want to fight us, my friend?' said the black boy. He slapped his fist in his hand and laughed. 'Defend the honour of your little ladybug.' He looked me hard in the eye. 'What you gotta say? Huh?'

'The ladybird's flown off,' I said, teeth clenched. 'I've got nothing more to say to either of you.'

'Ooooh, it sounds like he's a bit angry,' chided the black boy.

'Spot on,' I whispered.

'One more fucking word out of you,' shouted the white boy, prodding at me, 'one more bit of disrespect and I'll do you.' He glowered at me. 'Anything to say now, you fucker?'

I rolled my eyes at him and hunkered down miserably into my seat. The two boys turned around, laughing. I'd never felt more humiliated in my life.

BB and I had to get off at the next stop. Silence fell between us for a while as we walked back to the office.

'I feel humiliated,' I said.

'Why?' asked BB. 'At least you spoke to them.'

'But I didn't stand up to them!' I shouted. 'I was a coward, I backed down. They were just kids.'

'They were grown men with kids' brains,' said BB. 'And they might well have had weapons. You did what you could.'

I paused. 'And where were you, BB?'

'What's that supposed to mean?'

'You said nothing. That's not the BB I know.'

'You think you know everyone, new boy. That's your problem.' She stopped and steered me on to a patch of green, away from the busy pavement. 'You need to understand something, Jimmy. Ten years ago I'd have grabbed those boys by the ear and slapped them. But not now, sadly.'

She sat down on a bench and beckoned me to sit by her. A cluster of starlings were pecking around in front of us.

'Most of the nurses in our office live away from this area, Jimmy,' she said. 'Well, I don't. I live right in the heart of it and have done for years. It's rough and ready, but it's cheap, my kids are at school here, and I've grown fond of it. In mental health nursing we are advised to live away from our work . . . '

'In case you bump into clients?' I interrupted.

'Exactly that.' She turned to look at me. 'Well, one time I did bump into a client. It was unfortunate. He was in a state of psychosis and wanted to talk to me. I was in a hurry to get home. I tried to be polite but he followed me. He pushed me against a wall and hit me in the face.'

'Ouch, I'm sorry,' I said.

'It wasn't so bad,' BB shrugged. 'A couple of men came to help and I managed to get away. I only got a black eye but it shook me up. The client was sectioned the next day. I still know him. We get on fine.'

BB sighed and put her hands on her lap like a child about to say grace. 'Two years after that incident I got assaulted in a park. It was during an early morning jog. This time my attacker had a knife.' She paused and rubbed her forehead with her palms. 'I scratched and kicked the bastard and by some miracle got away with only a scar on my arm. The whole thing freaked me out though.'

'I'm not surprised.'

'They never found the guy,' BB said, kicking at a tussock of weeds by the bench. 'And since then I'm scared. Really scared. I used to be bold as brass, you know. Hell, I even broke up fights in pubs.' She grinned at the memory. 'I'm just as outraged as you about what happened on the bus. But I'm a mother now. I have a family. And, yes, I've lost my bottle. It's OK, mucking around with Barry in the dojo, but real aggro scares me.'

BB fumbled in her handbag, pulled out a strip of gum and began to chew. 'You know, new boy, last week an old man was beaten to death two streets down from where I live.' She frowned and gestured across the park. 'He was over eighty years old. A gang of hoodlums kicked him in the head for the fun of it.

So yes, Jimmy, I'm careful now. I live around here. Those boys on the bus live around here. I see shit happen all the time around here. And I'm scared now, so I no longer take action. I'm not proud of myself at all.' She nudged me gently on my arm. 'So I'm sorry I was quiet on the bus, but I hope you understand.'

'Of course, BB,' I insisted. 'You're bloody brave to still do the job you do. I've never been in a fight in my life. I've no right to moralise.'

'Don't be sorry, new boy. People need to stand up to boys like those ones on the bus. I'm sure they've got good reasons for being so nasty – drugs, poverty, abuse. Who knows? But that's no reason not to challenge them. You could have been tougher, but hey, you didn't completely cave in. That's a start.'

BB stood up from the bench and raised her face to the sun. Together we started walking back to the office.

'So then,' said BB, marching, as always, two steps ahead of me, 'now you know my Barry's Nose. When am I going to get to know yours, hey?'

Chapter 15

THE WISDOM OF SOLOMON

'No one ever says thanks! It's a disgrace, innit, Jimmy!'

Hadia was holding court outside the hospital. We were both drinking tea and looking out over a fountain filled with frothy water. Hadia had just started her placement on a ward with a dozen mentally unwell teenagers – I was soon due to join her – and it was clearly taking its toll on her. She had already decided mental health nursing was not for her.

'None of the kids have any manners, Jimmy,' she said, blowing on her tea. 'And one of them, this cocky bugger called Solomon,' she said furiously, 'he flipping called me Darth Vader because of my black headdress. And he gets away with it cos he's a bit mad, innit!'

I could understand Hadia's frustration. Children's nurses, like her, were used to being thanked for their actions on the wards by grateful families. Indeed, children's wards were usually brimming with gifts to the nurses – chocolates, flowers or 'You're an Angel' cards. In contrast, mental health wards were threadbare, often not a box of Maltesers or a bunch of carnations in sight.

This wasn't something I'd noticed until Hadia pointed it out. It didn't really bother me much. With mental health the thank yous were just more subtle – a smile, a wink, a 'cheers, Jimmy,' or even a 'sorry, mate' after an episode of verbal abuse. It just took a bit longer to build up trust than on children's wards.

'Calling me Darth Vader,' grumbled Hadia. 'The little flipping nutty little bugger, innit!' Her vocabulary was becoming richer by the minute.

'That's the thing I like about you, Hadia, you tell it like it is.'

But it wasn't the lack of thank yous or the Darth Vader jibes that was Hadia's problem. Bigger things were eating at her, as I discovered as our conversation progressed.

'I'm not as confident as you think, Jimmy,' she stressed, looking me hard in the eye. 'It's a problem for me. People think I can deal with anything. I'm not only a student nurse, you know.' She shook her head. 'Oh, no, my life is far more complicated than that!'

Hadia explained that she worked at her dad's shop at the weekends, and had fallen in love with a distant cousin whose family couldn't stand her. Oh, and she was also up to her neck in coursework.

'And then I'm called Darth Vader . . . ' Hadia's eyes welled. For someone who had just turned twenty she certainly had a lot on her plate.

I sipped my tea and waited for Hadia to compose herself, but then, in a torrent of choked-up emotion, she let it all out. She told me she had never been this stressed. In the past she had always achieved things so easily. But this course was just 'crazy, innit'. All her friends were doing subjects like media or economics and got loads of time off to have fun, but for Hadia it was all work, work, work.

Hadia took a deep breath and explained that last month a child she was nursing had died. A sweet little girl with sickle-cell anaemia – her system had just collapsed. Nothing to be done, nobody's fault, but she didn't pull through. At first Hadia was fine, said she could handle it. Then one morning at the local mosque she 'just lost it', had a panic attack and cried her heart out. She chose not to tell any family or friends because she thought a dead child was beyond their grasp. She told her mentor instead, who put her in touch with a psychotherapist. The therapist was sympathetic and told Hadia she had too much on her shoulders for her age, that a child's death would knock even the hardiest of nurses. She told Hadia to take some time off, and to cast off her 'I can deal with anything' front, or she'd never survive the course.

'She's right,' I said. 'Seeing a child die is as hard as it gets. You need to talk it through with someone.'

'It wasn't just the child, Jimmy.' Hadia stirred at her tea, momentarily lost in thought.

'On the tube home after the therapist's session,' Hadia swung her gaze back to me, 'I was reading a newspaper. It had a story about that crazy Muslim preacher with the hook on his hand. Abu whatshisname. The story was so one-sided, making out all Muslims are like him, innit.'

'Well, you haven't got a hook,' I said. 'Or an eye patch.'

She smiled, out of politeness rather than amusement.

'But it upset me so much, Jimmy,' she added. 'As if just by being a Muslim I'm an enemy. I think this hook man is a flipping idiot and hate being labelled with him. I love this country and I love Allah, too, but reading that article made me feel like I don't belong, so I just lost it – in front of everyone on the train. Everything just hit me at once – the dead child, my loneliness. I cried my flipping eyes out.'

'It's OK, Hadia, it's healthy to cry sometimes.'

'Not for me!' she snapped, then immediately put up her hand by means of apology. 'I'm sorry, Jimmy, I'm just so tired. I feel so out of tune with my friends. Working on wards, in the shop, writing essays, in love with someone I shouldn't be.' She rolled her eyes. 'Oh my word, I'm so sorry to spill my guts like this. The therapist told me it would help.'

I told her I thought the therapist was right – she had loads on her plate and a bit of time out from the course, maybe just a week or two, might be an idea. No shame in that.

'No flipping way, innit.' Hadia looked at me, incredulous. I was amazed how many times Hadia had said 'flipping' – she was turning into a genteel version of Gordon Ramsay. 'I've battled my way through this flipping diploma for almost three years, Jimmy. I absolutely have to make it. Make it for my family, for my faith, for myself. What did Mr Temple say: "That what makes you suffer makes you stronger!"'

'Sounds far too profound for Mr Temple.'

'Well, whoever it was, they were right. So no way will I pull out.' She smiled. 'You know in the first year Mr Temple once said to me when I was late for a lecture: "Hadia, you're all froth and no coffee".'

'Yeah, that sounds more like him.'

'It really hurt at the time. But when I saw him recently he told me I was "all coffee and no froth".'

'Coming from Mr Temple that's high praise,' I said. 'Next he'll be adding chocolate topping with a dash of nutmeg. You deserve it, Hadia, you really do.'

We talked for a while longer but soon Hadia had to rush off to catch a train to Birmingham. She planned to write an essay during the journey, work in her father's shop all weekend and return to the ward on Monday morning. I just hope someone thanked her for it.

I joined Hadia on the same ward a week later. By then she was painting a far rosier picture of the place. She had even started to warm to her one-time nemesis, Solomon, who had stopped telling her she looked like Darth Vader. I certainly got a good vibe about the placement from the start and was pleased to be finally working in child and adolescent mental health.

My mentor, Josie, was a soft-spoken woman in her forties, who often assigned me Solomon as one of my daily patients.

'Watch out, Jimmy,' joked Hadia on my first day. 'With me as Darth Vader he'll probably call you Gollum.'

In fact, Solomon proved to be the patient I enjoyed working with the most. He was a cocky, half-Mauritian boy and, two months shy of his eighteenth birthday, was the oldest on the ward. For all his flashes of anger and his inability to sit still, there was something exceptional about Solomon.

Short, dark, wiry and very bright, Solomon moved and talked as if always on a quest – to learn the *Guinness Book of Records* by heart, master a guitar chord, perfect a slam dunk. He could be hyper and lippy but also gentle, especially with the most vulnerable children on the ward – a weepy girl with anorexia called Jane, a permanently angry Somali youth called Sadik and a mournful boy called Ron, who had recently attempted suicide. Solomon would always draw these outsiders into his playful orbit, make them laugh and build their confidence.

When working with Solomon shifts tended to be action-packed. The two of us would ping-pong between his medication rounds, school classes, music therapy, basketball and IT sessions. It was by far the best ward I had worked on for keeping patients stimulated, a world apart from the often listless adult units.

My mentor, Josie, was always on the lookout for new activities. One morning she asked all the teenagers to build their own flying machines using only cardboard, tissue, string and glue. But then came the really tricky bit. They had to attach a cream egg to act as a pilot and make sure it didn't smash. Within an hour all the children had finished. One by one Josie, Hadia and I threw the different flying machines from a first-floor window. SPLAT! SPLAT! SPLAT! All the eggs scrambled on landing. Solomon's egg was last up. Incredibly it survived, cocooned in an ingenious, heavily padded cardboard parachute. The children all whooped with delight as it swooped safely to earth.

Solomon's mental quests were not only restricted to eggs and flying machines. He was also determined to find out more

about his mental illness and researched all his diagnoses doggedly. He accepted he was messed up: he'd got into a few fights,
self-harmed a bit (cut his arms, burnt his fingers) and smoked far
too much cannabis, which had led to him occasionally hearing
voices.

Solomon's mental illness had been diagnosed as onset schizophrenia. He lived in desperate poverty with his mini-cab-driving
Mauritian father, his mother having died of cancer a couple of
years ago. He spoke both French and English fluently.

Solomon's doctors were deliberating over whether or not his
past use of skunk (a potent form of cannabis) was at the root
of his current mental problems, even though it could not be
conclusively proved. It was worth looking into. As a student
nurse I had seen so many skunk-smoking clients who were
mentally unwell. Indeed, skunk made up 80 per cent of the cannabis seized in the UK.

On my second week I was flattered when Josie invited me
to attend Solomon's ward-round meeting. She said I could
tag along with her and the rest of Solomon's health care team.
The meeting had been specially requested by Solomon. He not
only wanted to challenge the medication he was receiving but
whether he was mentally ill at all.

The meeting took place in a large conference room to the side
of the ward. It had an executive look, with large pot plants,
minimalist paintings and plates of posh biscuits. Solomon's
psychiatrist, Dr Pinter, an imperious redhead with a cut-glass
accent, sat at the head of the table. Fanning out either side of her
were Solomon's social worker, his music therapist, Josie and me.
At the far end of the table sat Solomon, decked out in a dark
suit, and his father, the mini cab driver, a tiny, intense man in a
battered leather jacket.

Dr Pinter kicked off by explaining why, in her opinion,
Solomon needed to be on antipsychotic medication (quetiapine)

and a mood stabiliser (diazepam). She stressed he had self-harmed and heard voices and that to take him off medication, or worse, off the ward, was unthinkable.

Solomon listened patiently, at times nodding his head, at times shaking it.

'Dr Pinter,' he said, once she had finished. 'Please understand I respect your point of view. I know it takes a long time to train to be a psychiatrist and you know much more about mental illness than me.' Dr Pinter smiled in a self-satisfied manner. 'But I want to make clear I know my *own* mental state very well. And I don't believe I have schizophrenia.'

'That's because of your medication, Solomon,' Dr Pinter said firmly. 'If you came off it, you would relapse.'

'But the diazepam makes me feel silly and spaced out and the quetiapine makes me put on weight.' Solomon put up his hands in protest. 'I've read all about them on the internet. You could at least cut down my dose a bit and see how I do.'

'I'm afraid that's out of the question for now.'

Solomon breathed heavily and drummed his fingers on the table.

'My behaviour has been very good lately,' he said.

'You called one student nurse Darth Vader, Solomon – that's not good.'

'That was a joke, doctor. Please ask the others if I have been well behaved.' Solomon implored the other health professionals.

The social worker and the music therapist both agreed Solomon had made great progress over the last couple of months. Josie stayed quiet, so I mentioned that Solomon had been very generous to the other children during a recent game of basketball. He had patiently taught them how to shoot hoops. I also mentioned that Hadia had been under a lot of stress the day Solomon called her Darth Vader, and she now accepted the comment was a joke.

'To be fair, Dr Pinter,' said Solomon, 'you don't even know what mental illness I have.' This was true, his diagnosis had veered wildly over time. He had started off as a bog-standard dopehead (not the professional jargon), before being pigeon-holed with bipolar disorder and now schizophrenia.

'I don't think I'm mentally ill,' stressed Solomon. 'My mum died, my dad's been depressed. So yes, it's been a really tough time. Made me do stupid stuff, like smoke loads of skunk. The skunk made me hear weird voices now and then.' He rolled his eyes and pulled a stoned, hippy-like face. 'But I haven't smoked it for ages, and I won't go back to it. I know I've still got my troubles but I'm so much better than I was. Maybe I've just got a slight personality disorder or something.'

'Do you even know what personality disorders are, Solomon?' asked Dr Pinter.

'Sure, I've read about them. All the different types – border-line, schizo, and what have you. It's more to do with what's happened to you in your life, rather than your genetics. Like if you have been badly treated as a child, you might be very aggressive or very shy.' He tapped his forehead with a finger. 'I also know you often don't need medication, just therapy. I'd prefer that . . . '

'That's a very simple explanation of personality disorder,' butted in Dr Pinter. She really did have a wonderfully superior manner. 'Though it is possible you have schizo-affective dis-order – a cross between schizophrenia and mood disorder.'

'I know what it is,' said Solomon politely. 'And with respect, I'd like to stress again that nobody seems to really know what I've got.'

Solomon was well within his rights to emphasise this. Even in the nursing station every one of us had our own ideas.

'Mental illness is hard to pinpoint exactly sometimes,' said Dr Pinter in a tired voice. 'And life is unfair sometimes, Solomon.'

'I know life is unfair, doctor,' Solomon's voice had an edge of anger now. 'I read the other day that the 400 richest people in the world have more money put together than the poorest two billion. How nuts is that? Did you know that, Dr Pinter?'

'I'm not paid to know that. I'm paid to help you. I know you are very smart, Solomon but . . . '

'Did you know the Panama Canal opened on the day the First World War started, Doctor? Did you know that, hey?'

'Solomon . . . '

'Did you know that one in six of the long-term jobless are dead within ten years, Dr Pinter? Does it bother you that if you keep me in here I might become one of them?'

'Calm down, Solomon,' urged Josie. Solomon's father, until then impassive, put his arm round his son's shoulder to placate him.

'The doctor isn't listening to me,' Solomon protested. 'Just saying the same old stuff. I'm doing everything in my power to get better here. Music therapy, lessons, sport. I turn eighteen any minute, and I know adult wards are really bad compared to here. I'm not stupid. I want to make something of myself. Not be stuck in some ward, drugged up to my eyeballs. I went through a bad patch, but isn't that understandable given my situation?'

'You need to calm down, young man,' insisted Dr Pinter.

'I'd like to say something,' said Josie. Her voice was quavering with nerves.

'Go ahead, Josie,' said Dr Pinter sharply.

'Forgive me, doctor.' Josie raised her palms in a calming gesture. 'But I think Solomon is making some valid points. He is a smart young man who could do well given the chance. He has been trying very hard recently. Perhaps we could at least consider cutting his medication.' Josie was so nervous I feared she might dry up completely. 'I'm sorry, doctor. But I also think you have sounded a bit patronising towards him. That's why he's getting a bit angry.'

Dr Pinter looked like thunder. 'This is not the place for this now, Josie,' she said, barely containing her wrath. 'We need to make a unanimous decision and I'm convinced we must keep his medication as it is. So, are you with me or not?'

Josie had showed great bravery. She was a timid, non-confrontational person and had managed to fire a broadside at Dr Pinter. But her firepower was now spent. She nodded in agreement.

Solomon got up slowly, his face tight and inscrutable. He smiled, said 'thank you for nothing' and walked out. His father, unable to speak much English and ill at ease since the start of the meeting, scampered after him.

'Josie, we must keep up a united front,' snapped Dr Pinter, as soon as Solomon had left.

'Yes, doctor.' Josie's voice remained shaky. 'I'm just worried Solomon will struggle on an adult ward. He's done so well here. I fear he'll fall through the cracks between child and adult services. I've seen it before.'

'Yes, you've made your concerns quite clear, Josie.' Dr Pinter rapped her hands on the table. 'But I've made my decision and we must stick to it.'

'Yes, doctor.'

'Right then,' said Dr Pinter. 'That's it. End of meeting.'

I couldn't believe how cowed Josie was now. She was the same age as Dr Pinter, maybe older, with over a decade's experience in the nursing front line. In her career she had taken part in restraints, comforted murderers, witnessed suicides – things some psychiatrists might never do. But here in front of Dr Pinter she was quavering like a chastised schoolgirl.

Back in the ward that afternoon Solomon seemed surprisingly sanguine when I asked him how he felt.

'I'm not too worried to be honest, Jimmy,' he said. 'No way am I going to an adult ward – the thought scares the shit out of me. So I've no option. I'm out of here.' I didn't pay too much attention to his 'I'm out of here' comment at the time, thinking he was either joking or acting tough.

Later that morning Solomon took a cigarette break outside the ward. He left his bedroom window ajar with his coat perched on the ledge. When the escort nurse was distracted by a call on his mobile Solomon grabbed his coat and sprinted up the gravel drive. In no time he had disappeared into the busy streets.

The day after Solomon's escape Hadia and I returned to college for our final exams. I did my best to put the fact that Solomon was in serious trouble temporarily out of my mind and focus on my finals.

First up was the wretched drug calculation test. I wished Hadia good luck and split off to join Kiko and the rest of the mental health group in our corner of the exam hall.

The drug test was only ten questions, covering subjects that even if whispered in a thrillingly seductive accent by Penélope Cruz – 'milligrams of mercury, mi amor . . .' – would still sound deadly.

Three years ago a test like this would have brought me out in a cold sweat. I'd hated Maths at school, and it had taken me multiple efforts to pass my GCSE. All that needless algebra, those long equations, skills I knew I'd never use beyond the classroom. But, strangely, as a nursing student I had started to enjoy Maths calculations. Here, suddenly, was purposeful arithmetic, essential number crunching, so unlike the tortuous stuff I had wrestled with as a child.

Following the Maths test all of us frantically compared answers. Kiko and I were in synch with our sums, which boosted my spirits. We got a second chance with all our exams but fail again and then, kaput, the show's over. Three years flushed down the drain. It was always best to nail a nursing exam first time.

That afternoon we also took our final OSCE. Unlike the OSCE in the first year, when I had done 'the obs' on a bed-bound patient, the mental health OSCE involved no thermometers, blood pressure machines or 'Nellie the Elephant'. Instead, each of us had to teach a topic relevant to mental health to a first-year student. The topic given to me was 'substance misuse'. As I'd worked with several patients with drug- and booze-related problems, I felt confident I could pass. I was further fortunate to be teaching a student with an Oscar-winning 'I'm fascinated' look, even though she must have been bored rigid, having heard the same spiel dozens of times by then.

After it was over I felt a sudden sense of calm. We wouldn't hear the exam results for a month or so, but unlike previous exams I was quietly confident I'd bagged them both. We still had a dissertation and an end-of-year portfolio to hand in, plus I needed to clock up dozens more hours on placement with BB and the team – but, for all that, I knew qualification was finally in sight.

I was doubly chuffed when my mental health colleagues presented me with a post-OSCE birthday cake (bloody Facebook). Other than Kiko I didn't really know the group that well and felt bad I hadn't made more effort with them. They were a good bunch. As we all munched on the cake, for the first time in a long time, I felt at peace with the world.

'Jimmy,' shouted Vicky, who had also just finished her OSCE. I turned round and saw her running towards me, with Hadia and Coco hot on her heels. They looked like a nursing version of *Charlie's Angels*.

'Hey girls,' I said. 'Come and have some birthday cake. Where's Jana?'

'She didn't turn up for her exams,' said Vicky. 'None of us can get through to her on her mobile.'

'What? You've got to be joking!'

I pulled out my phone and tried her – the call went straight to the answering machine. Vicky said she'd also tried Facebook, but Jana had taken herself off the network.

'I've heard she's missed lots of placement shifts,' said Vicky, 'and moved out of the nursing halls.'

'But we're so near the end!' I shook my head in disbelief.

'It's weird her not turning up for finals,' said Hadia. 'Must mean she really has dropped out this time.'

'Let's all try to get in touch with her,' stressed Vicky. 'Jana's been with us from the start. It's the least we can do.'

I persistently phoned Jana over that weekend. When I finally did get through she sounded subdued. I told her a million reasons why she shouldn't quit the course but her mind was made up. We agreed to meet for a drink at Seamus's.

'I'm sorry, Jimmy, but I'm really out this time,' she said, sipping a Guinness. 'I've thought long and hard about it. I'm working as a nanny instead. I've got myself a man now, too.' She smiled. 'And, yes, before you ask, it was through internet dating.' She rolled her eyes. 'But I'm doing OK, Jimmy. I just didn't want the stress of being a nurse.'

'But that's three years down the . . . ' I started but dried up when she gave me a killer look.

'You've already had your say, Jimmy. So's Hadia, Vicky and Coco.'

'OK, OK, I'm not here to lecture you. You've clearly thought it through. But we'll stay in touch, right?'

'Of course,' she said. 'It's just every time I see any of you guys, I'll be ashamed. Be reminded that I flunked out.'

'You had valid reasons, Jana.' I wagged a finger at her. 'And by the way, we are capable of talking about things other than nursing, you know!'

'Really,' she said, laughing. 'But every single time we get together we always talk about nursing.'

'True,' I conceded. 'But we've had some good times, too, hey. Don't forget that.'

'I won't,' she said. 'Look, I'm sorry it hasn't worked out. I'll really miss you guys. At least everything I've learnt about kids will help me nannying.' She winked. 'I'll even know how to tranquillise any tricky ones.'

'Our loss is the nanny world's gain!' I said, and meant it.

After that Jana fell off my radar. We tried half-heartedly to stay in touch, but with placements and final deadlines looming, time was tight. Jana, too, was absorbed in another life.

I felt gutted Jana had quit in the closing months of the course and kicked myself that I hadn't been there for her. I'd been too wrapped up in my own orbit. She had been the star pupil of our group and I took it for granted she'd make it. How wrong you can be sometimes.

Jana also lost contact with Vicky, Hadia and Coco. We could understand why she had distanced herself from us, but it was still a blow. For me, Jana's friendship, support and piss-taking had been vital in getting me through this far. If I ever got my nursing degree, I decided, a lot of it was down to her.

Thankfully, there was some good news to soften the blow of Jana's departure when Hadia and I returned to the adolescent ward on the Monday after our finals.

As we all gathered for handover in the nurses' station Dr Pinter came in to announce that Solomon had phoned. He'd apologised for running away and was due back in an hour. We all let out a collective whoop of delight that he was safe. Josie dissolved into quiet tears. Dr Pinter gave her a brief, supportive squeeze on the arm and walked away.

On arrival at the ward Solomon made a beeline straight for Hadia. 'I'm so sorry I ever called you, Darth Vader,' he said, bowing in apology. 'I was playing around but I was very rude. You are a good person, Hadia. More like Princess Leia.'

'Oh, don't make me blush, Solomon,' Hadia replied. 'It's great to have you back, young man.' She nudged him on the arm. 'And get a haircut will you. You're beginning to look like Chewbacca!'

Chapter 16

AMONG THE ANGELS

Although I still needed to clock up time both on Solomon's ward and with BB, it was dawning on me that my student nurse journey was almost over.

It seems everyone makes a journey these days: *X Factor* contestants always blub about their journeys, as do master chefs and footballers. Even Tony Blair has called his autobiography: *A Journey*. Fair enough, he's taken most of us for a ride.

I'd forgotten a golden rule, though – that at the end of every journey you let down your guard. You think you are home and dry, on the cusp of glory, and at that precise moment, the gods of rum fortune shoot you out of the sky. It's happened since journeys began. Look at poor old Odysseus, perhaps the first great traveller; just when he was on the home straight his men were turned into pigs.

OK, it's fair to say a nursing degree is not on a par with battling storms, sea monsters and pig-making sorceresses, but I was still proud to have got this far. And Homer's advice in The Odyssey was still spot on more than two millennia later – the time for greatest vigilance really is at the voyage's end.

I'd survived adult, children's and mental health placements, Mr Temple's barbs, Mr Smith's fury, Jacko's fists, Joanna's hugs

241

and Jana's departure. I'd helped care for the best of patients and the worst of patients. I'd completed my final exams, served time at Holloway and now, incredibly, was finishing my final weeks on placement as a student nurse.

These placements were mostly with BB – flitting between the ward and the community. Back at the ward I was particularly pleased by Solomon's progress. Since returning from his ill-advised escape bid he'd been a star, attending all his classes, playing lots of sport and acting as a great role model to the other children. When Hadia occasionally came back for a shift, he'd call her 'Princess Leia', which always made her smile. Even Dr Pinter agreed to drop the dose of Solomon's medication – but still stuck firmly to her diagnosis of schizophrenia.

It wasn't long before Solomon was discharged and returned to his father's flat. But he still attended a day centre near the ward five times a week, where I met up with him for a game of basketball or football now and then. For all his new politeness, occasionally his gangland lingo surfaced, usually in the heat of a football tournament.

After one of his team missed a particularly easy open goal he shouted: 'Mate, I could have scored that with my dick!'

Other insults were aimed at referees, but always under his breath. 'That ref's such a wimp he'd step out of the shower to piss,' being one of his favourites. I reprimanded him, but couldn't resist a smile. Besides, these jibes were never vindictive. Solomon was also coming on leaps and bounds at the guitar, winning praise from his music teacher.

It was great to see Solomon making something of himself. To me, it proved there was a way forward for those who suffer mental illness. It showed that young people like Solomon could make friends, have a love life (he was dating a pretty girl with peroxide blond hair) and follow their dreams – he was keen to try for university, maybe pursue a career in sport or music. He hadn't needed to go on to an adult ward, hadn't fallen through the cracks. All the nursing team were hugely proud of him.

Back in the community BB got me to sit in on some therapy sessions with children who had committed crimes. Before I attended my first session BB took me along to the therapy team's monthly debating forum. Josie and Dr Pinter were in attendance, along with various psychotherapists, psychologists and family therapists.

If there was a noun to describe a group of therapists – in the same way we categorise a pride of lions or a gaggle of geese – I reckon an 'intensity of therapists' would be perfect. Therapists of whatever description do tend to be pretty intense. Considering they are all supposed to be chock-full of empathy for their fellow man, they are certainly capable of some spectacular fallings out with each other, too.

At this particular forum we were discussing how a bunch of largely middle-class health professionals such as us – doctors, therapists and a few nurses – could credibly empathise with people who lived in one of the poorest areas of the country. How could the likes of us possibly understand their concerns?

'I've occasionally been guilty of putting clients on a pedestal,' said BB, kicking things off. 'Sometimes their stories of abuse, or poverty, or heartache are so acute, so divorced from my own life, I don't feel qualified to treat them.'

'But our job is to be empathetic,' stressed Dr Pinter, with a toss of her ginger mane. 'Not to beat ourselves up with middle-class guilt.'

'Oh, I agree, Dr Pinter,' BB nodded. 'But don't tell me you've never felt out of your depth with some of your clients. That their stories haven't left you speechless, or unable to act as rationally as you'd like.'

'No, not really,' said Dr Pinter imperiously. She looked intense. 'I just try to be professional.'

'Me, too,' agreed another therapist with half-moon specs and a fledgling beard. 'Just because I didn't grow up in a council flat with an abusive father, doesn't mean I can't empathise with someone who did.'

'But I take BB's point,' said Josie, raising her hand gingerly. 'I'm a nurse, and I expect I'm the nearest to a working-class person here. I'm sometimes in awe of what clients have gone through. I think it's dishonest to say we are always detached.'

'But . . . ' said Dr Pinter.

'I'd like to make a further point,' interrupted BB, taking a sheet of paper out from her handbag. 'I've brought this list along.' She waved it at the group. 'It's a list of words we therapists have used in sessions over the last month.'

She perused the list and smiled. 'OK, how about – "bifurcation", anyone, or "somatic expression" or "cross transference". All fine for us, but for a client with little education these are complex terms.' She laughed. 'In fact, I had a good education and I still didn't understand half of them.'

Dr Pinter looked like thunder. 'I think it's all right to use difficult words as long as they are clearly explained,' she said. I admired her courage in owning up to using the word 'bifurcation'.

'I think we can explain something without using unnecessarily complex jargon,' replied BB. 'For an example, who here can describe Freud's terms: ego, superego and id? Surely very tricky to sum up for anyone not in the mental health game.'

BB's challenge reminded me of a documentary I had seen recently where a group of top financial experts had been asked to describe what a 'derivative' is. Some bumbled away in incomprehensible City speak, others dried up and some, probably because they had no idea, refused. I've never understood what a derivative is, and was left none the wiser. If some of the world's leading financial brains couldn't help me out I wonder who could.

'The way I remember Freud's id, ego and superego,' said Dr Pinter, rising to BB's challenge (she certainly wasn't lacking guts), 'is by thinking of a horse, a chariot driver and the chariot driver's father.'

Blimey, I thought, the subconscious meets *Ben Hur.* Dr Pinter took a deep breath, and composed herself. She looked as if she was about to perform a difficult yoga move.

'The horse is the id,' she began. 'The instinctive spirit, where any impulse is acted on. Like when we are very young, if we want food, we scream. Is that clear?' We all nodded. 'The chariot driver is the ego, the rational part of you that takes responsibility for your own actions, makes you rein in your horse.' She pulled on an imaginary set of reins. 'And, finally, the chariot driver's father is the superego, the one who helps point out mistakes, provides a moral compass, advises whether to act more with id or with the ego.'

'How about the horse?' said BB. 'Does it even have an ego? Let alone a superego?' This was harsh. Dr Pinter's description hadn't been bad – I understood more about Freud now, well, more than I did about derivatives anyway.

'The horse is a representation of id, not ego . . . ' Dr Pinter started. 'Oh, never mind. I'd never describe this sort of stuff to a client anyway.'

'All I'm saying is that as health professionals we should try to keep things simple,' said BB, taking a pen out of her top pocket.

'You know something,' BB waved the pen in the air, 'NASA once spent millions of dollars designing a pen that would work in space.' She now pulled out a pencil from her pocket and held it up. 'The Russians just used a pencil instead. They kept it simple. Sometimes we should learn to do the same.'

And then, just as I was steering my own chariot into the final straight, the wheels came off . . .

It was during my initial day of therapy sessions with youth

offenders that I foundered. The therapist was a calm, softly spoken Afro-Caribbean woman called Gwen, whose gentle manner helped tease out information from the various children.

First up was fifteen-year-old Ghafor, a nervy, stutter-prone Afghan boy with gelled hair. He'd seen both his parents and elder brother gunned down by the Taliban, and later fled the country smuggled in the back of a truck. After a scary and exhausting overland journey he made it undetected into the UK, and stayed with an uncle, who worked all hours as a mechanic. With no one to properly care for him, Ghafor had got in with a gang of older boys and had started to take drugs – mostly crack. He'd been with his gang when they assaulted a rival gang member and nearly beat him to death. Ghafor had not been part of the attack but had done nothing to intervene.

The interview was conducted with an Afghan interpreter, and Ghafor often became tearful.

'My whole life has been full of fear, of violence,' he told us. 'I have nothing to live for. I'm so unhappy. I don't know what to do.'

The next session was with foppish, well-spoken seventeen-year-old Hugh, who had excelled at school, had loads of friends and a happy relationship with his parents and siblings. But a year ago Hugh's grades had slumped and he'd slowly become surly and combative. Then he'd started stealing things from home. It turned out he'd been smoking huge quantities of skunk, and was then caught selling it.

Hugh's father, a tall, bird-like man with a kind face, couldn't understand. 'Our son has changed,' he said. 'We love him so much, but he is not the same boy as he was. It's as though he's lost all the warmth and fun he had inside of him.'

There was a time, before I began nursing, when I thought legalising cannabis might be a good idea – let people make their own mind up, said my free-spirited side. Others thought the same and in 2004 cannabis was downgraded to Grade C status.

I was proved completely wrong and I'm glad to say, due to mounting evidence that the drug is harmful to mental health, especially to those under eighteen, it is now Grade B once again.

When Hugh left the therapy session for a toilet break, his father admitted: 'I smoked cannabis back in the 1970s, but this skunk stuff is toxic in comparison.'

His point was spot on. The 'peace and love' dope of the hippy period had given cannabis a benign image, but the skunk of today was increasingly proving to be something much more sinister.

I felt for Hugh's father. His once talented and loving son was now overweight, grouchy and liable to the shakes. He had also started hearing voices – possibly meaning he was in the grip of early onset schizophrenia. This golden boy's future, once so bright, was now clouded by the spectre of medication and mental institutions: all perhaps sparked by Hugh firing up, in a moment of innocent fun-seeking, that first spliff.

The day rolled on, the tragedies unrelenting. There was a fourteen-year-old girl who had started a house fire to hurt a love rival; and a boy who had assaulted his cousin with a knife. Finally we saw a teenager who had tried to force his younger sister to perform oral sex on him. The boy, who was wearing a jumper the colour of porridge, studded with cigarette burns, told us his stepfather had sexually abused both him and his sister. By the end of the grimmest of sessions I just wanted to find the stepfather and shake him: 'Stop! Stop this dreadful cycle! Say sorry and just leave them alone!'

I came out shell-shocked. I could now understand BB's assertion that sometimes health professionals put certain types of client on pedestals and feel ill-equipped to cope with the sheer horror of their experience. For me, this was only exacerbated when working with these children, who were not only the victims of crime or abuse, but sometimes, confusingly, the perpetrators, too.

I spent the rest of the week observing and, at times, contributing to the therapy sessions with the young offenders. It didn't get any better; each day I came out feeling sick in my stomach. I also gained a new respect for therapists. These were not the sort of flaky 'make yourself rich/happy/thin/sexy' therapists, they were doing their very best to help the most vulnerable children in society. It was a bloody hard job. I have to confess that hearing all the children's tales of unhappiness – even if only for a week – had started to corrode my sense of hope. I admired those who could listen and empathise on a daily basis.

That Friday evening I met up with Hadia at a local cafe, near to where we were both working. She was uncharacteristically quiet. The cafe was about to close and we took our takeaway coffees to a patch of scrappy parkland and sat with our faces to the evening sun. We were silent for a while and then Hadia told me that Solomon was dead.

The evening before, he'd got back in with some of his old gang members and gone for a joyride. The car had flipped and Solomon, who was in the passenger seat, was killed outright. The others had received minor injuries but were now all out of hospital. All of them were believed to have been drunk.

'I was going to phone you, Jimmy,' said Hadia. 'But I thought I should tell you face to face. I know you two got on well.'

That evening, for the first time since starting nursing, I needed, rather than fancied, a drink. I propped up my local bar and sank a couple of pints. Solomon had been the beacon of hope, the one who slipped the statistics, the one who was going to make it. I laughed bitterly when I remembered him telling me: 'Us nutters are all creative geniuses, Jimmy. Beethoven, Kurt Cobain. I've read about them. You wait, I'll soon be famous.'

I got back to my flat, kicked at some furniture, and, unable to sit still, went out for a walk around the local park. The summer light was fading fast, but there were still several people eating, drinking, kicking footballs, hurling frisbees. After a while I calmed down a bit, let the violence and despair drain out of me. I sat on a bench looking out over a pond, studded with algae and reeds. The odd duck was gliding about.

After a long time I took out my mobile and punched the speed dial.

'Hello!'

'Poppin, is that you? It's daddy.'

'Daddy, you sound funny. Are you coming to babysit?'

'I'm in England, Pops, you know that. But I'll come and see you soon, I promise. How are you?'

And then she was off. Poppin was either chatty on the phone or didn't say a word. Tonight she was Miss Chinwag. She told me she had won a swimming tournament, that she wasn't learning ballet any more (the teacher was 'silly') and, oh yes, there was a sleepover at a friend's house at the weekend. What happened, I thought? She sounds like a teenager already. She chatted happily on until the line began breaking up.

'I can't wait to see you, Pops. I love you.'

'I love you, dad.'

And then she was gone, a faint hiss was all that was left on the line. I leant back on the bench. There was a smell of blossom in the air. It was dark now, the night sky a canvas of faint, luminous pinpricks.

'I love you,' I thought. They have to be the most overused, undervalued, maudlin, manipulative and insincere trio of syllables of all time. And yet, how dreadful it was that some of the men, women and children I had nursed over these last three years had never heard them. Because just once in a while 'I love you' lives up to its promise, hits the mark, bursts the poison and swells the heart – a talisman to stave off all harm.

Soon after this I sent an email to Kay in Mexico asking her when she was launching the street child project.

249

I got an immediate reply.

Any minute, Jimmy. Are you having second thoughts, amigo? I'll send you more details. Please come, even if only for a while! You'd be much closer to Poppin too!

'I'm ready to tell you my Barry's Nose, BB,' I said, as we sat writing up notes in her office. She paused and looked over her glasses at me.

'I'm all ears.'

'I don't think I'm cut out to be a nurse.'

'What?' shrieked BB. 'Why on earth not? This is so sudden.'

'It's not a knee-jerk reaction, BB,' I stressed. 'It's something I've come to realise over time.'

I explained about how much the child therapy sessions had got to me, followed by the knock-out blow of Solomon's death. I explained how I didn't enjoy the intense analysis of clients, or indeed myself. I explained that I felt medication was often given out too freely to mentally unwell children. I explained how even when working on the children and adult wards in my first year, I didn't have the natural, selfless qualities of many nurses. Sure, I had performed well enough, but I didn't have that indefinable gift I'd seen in others – in Vicky, Jana, Hadia, Kiko and many of my mentors – that willingness to give themselves 100 per cent to others.

'You're no angel, Jimmy,' said BB. 'But you'd still cut it as a nurse. And remember, it's a job for life.' She paused and studied her pen. 'But I see where you are coming from. You are clearly a person who likes results. You're not very patient. The wards might not be for you.'

'That's my problem,' I explained. 'I'm selfish. Most nurses don't need that, they are just happy to try to help.'

'Have you thought about being a youth support worker?' said BB. 'You could act as a mentor in a youth offending team, or

something like that. You'd be dealing more with the empowering and recreational stuff than the analytical or medicinal.'

'Sounds good.'

'I think you're like me, new boy,' said BB. 'You're fed up
with everyone banging on about the youth of today being useless. I think you're idealistic with your gardening, sports, activities and all that, but you might just do some good.'

I told BB that I'd recently read a book she'd recommended
called *Man's Search for Meaning* by Viktor Frankl. In it Frankl
writes about his time in a concentration camp during World
War Two. After his release, having withstood the most dehu-
manising treatment, Frankl decides that our main human drive
in life is not pleasure (as Freud thought) or power (as several
others thought) but meaning. In today's 'I want it all' society his
message seemed particularly relevant. I explained all this to BB.

'I think new skills help give a client, especially a child, a sense
of worth,' I said. 'Therapy and medication are important, of
course, but don't by themselves lead to meaning.'

'Phew, new boy, you're getting deep,' BB said, prodding me
with her pen. 'You clearly need to make a decision.'

'What do you think, BB?'

'I think you are a pain in the butt, Jimmy' she said. 'Who cares
what I think? You've got to decide. All I'll say is this. You've
got to do something that blows the wind up your trousers.' She
flicked her own skirt to demonstrate. 'Do something that fires
you up. Have you heard of the boiling-frog lesson?'

'Boiling frog?' I shook my head.

'Scientists have discovered that frogs have odd nervous systems
that react very slowly to change.' She pretended to pick up a frog,
using a stapler as a substitute. 'So if you sit a frog in a pan of water
and slowly heat it, the wretched thing will stay where it is until
it burns up.' She gave me a knowing look. 'So, new boy, choose
something you really want to do, or in a decade or so, you'll be
boiled, too.' She smiled at me. 'So what do you reckon?'

'I think I might go to Mexico for a few months.'

'Mexico. As in big hats and tequila. That Mexico?'

'No, BB. As in berets, croissants and vin rouge. Of course that Mexico.' I explained to BB what I wanted to do in Mexico, how it would take me closer to Poppin, how Kay's project excited me. How I hoped my training would help with the various problems I'd encountered in working with the street children, and with Kay's planned health clinic. How I spoke dodgy Spanish.

'Mexico!' BB fanned her face with a notepad and gave me a hard stare. 'Oh, God, new boy, I can see you're not joking. The first student I mentor, and he rides off into the sunset in a bloody sombrero. What about all your training?'

'I'll come back soon,' I said. 'But kick-starting the Mexico project will be a great experience. Then I can come back and do youth mentoring or work with mentally ill adolescents. Maybe set something up.'*

'Something stimulating,' said BB, rolling her eyes. 'Well, I suppose you've been OK, new boy, earned your spurs – you'll probably need a set of those in Mexico.' She shook her head. 'Man oh man, Mexico. Phewey. At least you're planning on coming back. I'd prefer you to start in the NHS, but being as you're already an old geezer, and it takes you nearer to your daughter and . . . Mexico.' She tut-tutted and punched me on the arm. 'Adios, you mad bugger.'

At the graduation ceremony I had my picture taken with Vicky, Hadia and Coco.

'I'm going to call this photo 'The Survivors',' said Coco, as we grinned and held up our mortar boards.

---

*In the joyous but unlikely event I make any royalties from this literary endeavour – my sister's book club means sales just might hit double figures – they will go towards helping adolescents with mental illness and/or substance misuse problems within the UK.

Vicky and Coco had both quickly found jobs on paediatric wards. Coco planned to work in the UK for another decade and then take her skills back to Africa, while Vicky was keen to cut her teeth in London-based hospitals. Hadia had secured a job in Birmingham, not nursing, but working with autistic children. She still worked in her father's shop at the weekends, and was dating her distant cousin. They all seemed very happy.

As we were saying our goodbyes and promising to stay in touch, Mr Temple walked over. It was hard to recognise him, dressed in his academic finery. He wore a saffron-coloured hat that made him look like some kind of Ruritanian grandee.

'Nice look, Mr Temple,' said Vicky. 'It suits you.'

'Well, well, well . . . ' he said, eyeing us in our robes. 'Three years ago I never thought you lot stood a chance. Especially you, Jimmy. But, as Einstein said: "If at first the idea is not absurd then there is no hope for it." You lot proved me wrong. You made it.'

I smiled. 'You made it.' From Mr Temple this was the equivalent of a hearty bear hug. I quickly banished this thought from my mind.

'Excuse me, but I've got to head back now,' Mr Temple told us. 'Interviewing a fresh bunch of recruits. Good luck to you all.'

He smiled that familiar menacing smile and glided off into the crowd. Now we were no longer his students, he was clearly hungry for fresh blood. I'd miss the old boy despite all the initial terror he stirred up in us. I thought back to that first interview with him, and poor Elsa reduced to tears. Elsa would be older now – I hoped she'd gone back for another shot at becoming a children's nurse. Maybe she was even one of Mr Temple's interviewees that afternoon.

Having handed back my graduation robes I met up with Kiko for a final drink at Seamus's. He had secured a job with the prison service, just as he'd wanted.

'I'm made up, man,' he said. 'Can't wait to get started. It will provide real stability for my family.'

Kiko told me that most of our mental health colleagues had landed jobs too, some in acute wards, some in rehab centres and one or two in the community. A couple of others had decided to carry on studying, Nicola to gain a degree in psychology, and Joe to qualify as a cognitive behavioural therapist.

It seemed none of us regretted our three years.

'So you're off to Mexico, bro!'

'Yes, I leave in a couple of weeks.'

'Whatever you do, don't get put in jail there,' said Kiko, slapping my back. 'I've heard they are some of the worst.'

'Not on my to-do list, Kiko.'

'Well, in my community in Africa we have a saying for good luck. It translates as something like "up the arse of a crocodile".'

'No wonder Senegal never win at football!'

We gave each other a slap on the back. 'Be good, Kiko – I hope you're a prison governor next time I see you.'

'Sure, bro. Don't forget to send me a postcard.'

The following weekend Jake, Bill and I were sitting in Bill's country garden drinking cider. We had just played a game of rounders with Bill's children and were sweating and out of breath from all the charging around. Bill's wife Ingrid was now packing the children off to bed. It was the first time the three of us had been together since Jake's leaving-do more than eighteen months earlier.

We had lots to celebrate. Bill had become a father again, Jake and Anna had fixed a date to marry next year and I had qualified as a nurse.

'I can't believe it,' said Bill, as we looked out across his overgrown lawn. 'One of you in Spain, and another off to Mexico.' He raised his hands up in the air. 'So much for our friends forever, band of brothers talk.'

'We'll soon both be back, Bill,' said Jake, slugging on a bottle of Magners. 'Besides, you bloody started it by moving here – commuter land. What was all that about?'

Bill told us he had moved to the country for his wife and children, but principally to be near his mother who was in a neighbouring nursing home. I knew Bill adored his mum. She had brought up Bill and his two brothers single-handedly. Bill's father had done a bunk and run off with another woman when Bill was a toddler.

'Mum's got really bad dementia now,' said Bill. 'She's often out of it, doesn't know who I am.' He paused and turned his face to the fading sun. 'Do you think they'll find a cure for dementia, Jimmy? I keep reading these articles in the papers and hoping.'

I told Bill that dementia-related drugs were improving all the time and that brain scans were getting increasingly sophisticated, but there was still a long way to go.

'The brain is so mindboggling,' said Jake. 'It's hard to believe we'll ever fully understand it.'

'I agree, mate,' replied Bill. 'I mean, some organs are so simple in comparison. Look at the heart – it's really just a pump, or the bladder, just a bag.' Bill put his hands on his forehead. 'But the brain. The bloody brain is still such a mystery.'

'Like a haggis stewing in strange chemicals,' said Jake. 'It's just so amazing, so weird.'

I tended to agree, at least with the 'amazing' and the 'weird', if not the 'haggis' bit. In recent years, thanks to scanning, we really did know much more about the brain – the synapses, the neuro-transmitters, the frontal lobe. But would we ever really know the brain's innermost secrets, I wondered. Would we know what makes us buy a season ticket for Sheffield Wednesday, or a Smart car, or a Big Mac or take up military fitness?

'At least Mum's standard of care at her home is good,' said Bill, frowning. 'But it might be closed due to NHS cuts. It would be completely crazy. The nurses are fantastic, Jimmy.'

I was glad to hear this. Over the past three years I had met some of the very best of nurses. Of course there were a few like Lord Mancroft described – jaded, rude – but considering their hours, their wages and their responsibility levels, the lion's share of my colleagues had been inspirational and I felt honoured to have worked among them. Yes, I know that sounds naff, but I don't care because it's true.

What upset me was that some of these nurses wanted out. One long-serving ward sister was about to throw in the towel because she was upset at spending all her time in meetings rather than with patients. Another nurse, who had returned to England after having worked abroad for a decade, said the NHS was now unrecognisable to her, with patient care being eclipsed by paperwork. It was hard for me to make comparisons after only three years as a student nurse but it saddened me the NHS seemed to be haemorrhaging some of its finest.

'The thing is,' Bill continued his quiet rant, 'I think Mum's home may be replaced by one of those stupid polyclinics. Her doctor said they are the future.'

'God help us,' I said.

These proposed all-singing, all-dancing polyclinics – huge hospitals supplying all medical services under one roof – sounded good on paper. But it would also mean some patients travelling for miles if their local services were shut down to make way for them. I feared they smacked too much of medical supermarkets: three-for-two deals are fine for pizzas, but surely not patients.

'Yeah, right on, comrade,' said Jake. 'They sound far too Orwellian. They'll wipe out all the small health trusts.'

'So what's the answer, Jimmy?' asked Bill.

I had no magic answers. It was pretty obvious lots of NHS money did go to waste, whether on polyclinics, lawsuits, sick days or chocolate Hobnobs eaten by groups of obscure health tsars. Oh, and flawed, vastly expensive computer modernisation schemes: almost all my patient notes over the last three years had been written by biro.

Yet, despite all this, and the fact that the NHS now boasted privately owned coffee shops and newsagents, privately employed cleaners and catering services, and Himalayan parking fees, it still managed to provide free health care to a nation. Surely, for all its faults, this in itself was a small miracle. Enough for it to retain its national treasure status.

Early in my training I realised the great behemoth that is the NHS is continually mocked by all those who work for her. Indeed, NHS staff like nothing better than a good rant – *oh, the bloody doctors/nurses/managers/patients/hours/wages/red tape/ creosote-flavoured coffee*. It doesn't matter who – matrons or midwives, cleaners or clinicians, techies or therapists, nurses or neurosurgeons, social workers or students (especially students) – we are all guilty.

But the NHS also inspires the greatest of loyalty. Like supporters of a much loved but down-on-its-luck football team (and I should know being a Sheffield Wednesday fan) we moan and tut-tut at our players' faults, but heaven forbid anyone who dares sneer too harshly – hands up Lord Mancroft – as then we will defend her with all our might.

'The NHS can't be all bad, Bill,' I said. 'Even Obama wants to copy the good bits of it over in America. We just need to stop wasting money, need to prioritise services.'

'Maybe the NHS could save money by axing inessential things,' said Jake. 'Like tonsil operations. Or Viagra.'

'Viagra,' stammered Bill. 'Oh, no! Give me a few more years and I'll be crying out for the stuff.'

We all laughed, three old school friends joking around with each other, something we'd been doing for more than twenty years now. Back in our teens we might have been discussing sex and drugs and rock'n'roll, now it was more likely to be parents/ wives/children, Omega-3 oils and the genius of Terry Wogan.

'I'd give up all the Viagra in the world just to find a cure for Mum,' said Bill, suddenly pensive. 'I can't believe I'm losing her. I owe that woman everything. She's my angel.'

Perhaps all three of us had our angels, I decided. Bill's mother had led him to the English boondocks, Anna's siren-call had enticed Jake to Spain and Poppin was now beckoning me across the Atlantic.

We all sat in silence scanning the horizon. A couple of yellow butterflies fluttered in the breeze. Bill's barbecue made sizzling noises and filled the air with delicious smells. I felt utterly relaxed, happy to be among old friends high on cider and sunshine. It was Jake who broke the spell.

'To your mum, Bill!' he blurted, suddenly raising his bottle.

'Yes, to angels!' Bill agreed, as we clanked our drinks together. 'And us devils they have to put up with!'

But there are many different kinds of angels.

About a week before I was due to fly to Mexico I was walking with Jake through the town centre. It was Saturday afternoon and the streets were teeming.

'Jimmy!' I heard a shout. I turned round and saw Joanna running towards me. It gave me a jolt seeing her so out of context – it had been a while since her hugging incident with BB, Dougal and me. But then I remembered she often got leave in the afternoons to do her shopping.

She'd put on some make-up and a smart new wig, with dark rather than fair hair. She'd also lost some weight and looked rather elegant.

'Hey, Joanna,' I said. 'You look great.'

I wondered what Jake would make of her. He remained in the background, smiling politely when Joanna looked at him. It was rare I bumped into clients, let alone while I was with a friend.

Joanna told me she was doing some computer lessons and had completed a diet – 'I breakfast like a queen, lunch like a princess and dine like a pauper, Jimmy!' She was pulling her life around. When she asked me what I'd been up to, I saw no reason to stay mum, now I was no longer working with her. I mentioned my graduation and the fact I was going to Mexico.

'Wow, well if you're going to Mexico, can I give you a hug?' said Joanna. 'A farewell hug from your little angel Joanna.' I burst out laughing, a combination of mirth and embarrassment. Oh, why not, I thought. I spread my arms and we gave each other a long, lung-suffocating hug, as the crowds navigated their way round us.

'And can I give your friend a hug, too?' she asked. 'He's much better looking than you.'

'Of course you can,' said Jake, rising to the occasion, and putting his arms towards her.

'I'll be your angel, too,' she said, as she enveloped Jake tight in her arms. I saw him turn a light shade of puce.

'See you then, Joanna,' I said, after all the embracing was done. 'You take care.'

'Remember, boys,' she said, readjusting her wig and blowing a kiss. 'I'm your guardian angel.'

'Who was that?' asked Jake. 'Someone from work? A friend of your mum or something? She's lovely, a right laugh.'

I was a bit taken aback by Jake's observation, and at first thought he was joking. I was about to tell him that Joanna was a client, give him some background – her mental illness, her substance misuse – but something stopped me. To him she was clearly just Joanna, a lovely, warm, funny and very tactile woman: why change that?

'Like she said, mate,' I replied, 'she's an angel.'